CROW MEDICINE

JANE RAY'S
WILDLIFE RESCUE SERIES

CROW MEDICINE

DIANE HAYNES

Walrus Books, an imprint of Whitecap Books

Edited by Sonnet Force
Proofread by Marilyn Bittman
Photo of Mouse by Don Haynes
Cover and interior design by Five Seventeen
Illustration by Five Seventeen
Typeset by Mark Macdonald and Michelle Mayne

Printed and bound in Canada

Library and Archives Canada Cataloguing in Publication
Haynes, Diane
    Crow medicine / Diane Haynes.
    (Jane Ray's animal rescue series ; 2)
ISBN 1-55285-806-5
ISBN 978-1-55285-806-6
    1. Crows--Juvenile fiction. I. Title. II. Series: Haynes, Diane.
    Jane Ray's animal rescue series ; 2
    PS8615.A85C76 2006   jC813'.6   C2006-900697-0

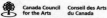

Canada Council   Conseil des Arts
for the Arts   du Canada

The author acknowledges the support of the Canada Council for the Arts.

The publisher acknowledges the support of the Canada Council for
the Arts, the British Columbia Arts Council and the Government of
Canada through the Book Publishing Industry Development Program
(BPIDP). Whitecap Books also acknowledges the financial support of the
Province of British Columbia through the Book Publishing Tax Credit.

Crow Medicine is dedicated to the staff, board, and volunteers of the WRA.

DISCLAIMER

CONTENTS

Prologue   11

1   All That Glitters   17

2   Corvophobia   27

3   Flory Delivers a History Lesson   34

4   West Nile Virus   41

5   Scapegoat   51

6   Cedars Mediterranean Café   58

7   Councilors' Haunt   66

8   Early Morning Visitor   74

9   The Crone   80

10   Bird Brain   88

11   Crow Medicine   98

12   Dirty Dancing   111

13   The Last Flight of Corvus   118

14   Stardust   128

15   Coffee Break   138

16   Shoot the Messenger   149

17   Flying Lessons   156

18   UHI   160

19   A Murder of Crows   167

20   Animal Rights . . . and Wrongs   172

21   Sick as a Dog   189

22   The Messenger and the Message   208

23   As the Crow Flies   221

24   No Word for Goodbye   238

25   Crow's Highway   245

26   A Night in the Crow's Nest   262

27   Leave It to Beaver   267

28   Jane Learns to Fly   273

29   Emergency Procedures   278

30   I Need a Vacation   291

31   Connect the Dots   295

32   Dinner Date   309

33   New Menus for Cedars   315

34   A Taste of Their Own Medicine   319

35   Amy Takes Orders   323

36   Take-Out and Delivery   328

37   Phoenix   330

     FLORY'S FILES   344

     ACKNOWLEDGEMENTS   348

     A NOTE FROM THE AUTHOR   351

What idea of order do I have that it
must exclude a starling, crow, or squirrel?

—Patrick Lane
There Is A Season: A Memoir

PROLOGUE

THE DEAD CROW lay in the middle of the curb lane, a small black stillpoint in the blur of morning rush hour. Its head faced forward with the traffic, lifeless wings flapping as though for takeoff each time a car sped over the little body. Instinctively, Jane slammed on her brakes, skidding to a stop in the center lane and making a long line of enemies behind her. Horns blared, windows were rolled down, and voices were raised, but all Jane could hear was the caahing of crows circling overhead, and her own blood pounding in her ears.

They'd stop if it was a human being, she thought, her hands strangling the steering wheel as cars continued to speed over the crow. *Or a dog.*

At a break in oncoming traffic, Jane spun left into the lower lot at Cedar's Ridge Senior Secondary and jammed her car into a free stall. Popping the trunk, she pulled gloves on, grabbed a towel and a plastic sack, then made her way carefully across four lanes of traffic to the sidewalk closest to the crow.

It was 8:00 a.m., the sun was already high in the sky and warm on Jane's shoulders, and a soft breeze blew through bright new leaves waving from the treetops above. The branches were thick with loud black birds, crows already at odds with the day. They called to her in insistent voices, almost in words. Jane lifted her face to the sky and called back, "I'll get him as soon as it's safe." *Crazy teen crushed in traffic rescuing dead crow*, she muttered to herself, shaking her head. The whizzing of cars whipped her long, dark hair wildly about her face, completing the picture.

Jane glanced left at the unbroken line of approaching cars, and then down at the crow. It was small. *Juvenile*, she thought. *His first spring. And his last.* The crow winked at her. She cried out. A car sped over the bird, lifting its wings again in that awful mockery of flight. Time slowed. Her blood roared in her ears. Road and trees and cars and school undulated as if underwater. *Juvenile*, Jane thought, her heart pounding. *Can't fly yet. Fledgling. Not dead. A fledge. Alive! He's alive!*

"He's alive!" Jane yelled the words out loud. She stepped off the curb, holding her left hand out like a traffic cop, and stared the next driver in the eye: "*Stop!*" The car skidded and swerved to avoid hitting her, and for the second time that morning, traffic outside Cedar's Ridge High came to a blaring standstill. Jane ignored the horns and bent over the crow. It turned its head toward her and blinked.

Jane tossed her towel over the small body and scooped him up off the road. In seconds, she was back at her car, trembling, her small bundle warm in her hands. As she reached for the kennel she always kept in her trunk, she realized the caahing of the other crows had gotten louder. Glancing up, she saw the lot of them, having abandoned the shelter of the trees, circling directly above her car. *He belongs to them*, she thought. *He's someone's child.*

Without thinking why, she raised the wrapped crow aloft above her head and made a promise: *If we can heal him, I'll bring him back here and release him to you.*

Minutes later, Jane pulled into the gravel parking lot at the Urban Wildlife Rescue Center. Hurrying into the reception area with the kennel, she called to Evie in the examination room, explaining between gulping breaths what had happened.

Evie Jordan emerged from the exam room, her normally cheery face grim. "Why did you bring him here, Jane?" Her words rang with accusation.

Stunned, Jane struggled for words. "Because . . . well, because you always know what to do!" What was up with Evie? She stared at the senior staffer, hoping something in her expression would provide a clue to her bizarre response.

Evie shook her head, scowling hard, and reached for the kennel containing the fledgling crow. Silently, she turned her back on Jane and made as if to disappear into the exam room.

"Hey, Evie!" Jane called after her, alarmed now. "What's going on? Is he going to make it? I'd like to be the one to release him, back where I got him. His family was . . . I mean, do you think . . . ?"

Evie turned slowly back to face Jane. She looked terribly sad. "Oh, Jane, didn't you know?" Jane shook her head, suddenly afraid. "All the crows are dying this year."

And before Jane could respond, Evie stepped into the exam room and pulled the sliding door closed.

"No!" Jane woke herself up with a yell. Her heart was pounding and her breath came in ragged gasps. Minnie mewed and stretched herself to twice her normal length, unwilling to leave the warmth of the bed. Sweet Pea leapt quietly to the floor and padded out of the room. Jane scrubbed her hands over her face, willing herself into the present. Remnants of her dream hung all around her, soft and black as crows' feathers, dangerous. *Where am I? What day is it? What's wrong?*

She turned her head to the right and opened an eye. 7:52. Thursday. May. School. No, something else. Signals with Amy and Flory! Missed them. Late. Late! Her weekly volunteer shift at the wildlife center. Eight minutes til it started. Late. She was going to be late.

Jane took a moment to breathe in the warm, lake-scented air wafting in through the big picture window. Sunlight beamed in wide swaths through the tops of the tall cedars surrounding the Ray home and landed in bright gold patches on her bookcase, the hardwood floor, Minnie's upturned tummy. *So glad it's a sunny day*, she thought, still half-tangled in her dark dream. Scooping up the little gray tabby, she kicked off the covers and hit the ground running.

Fifteen minutes later, she was backing up the long driveway, cats fed, banana scarfed, hair dripping, clothes askew. She rolled down the windows to let in the warmth of the sun and cranked the radio, bouncing in time to a dance tune, still trying to shake the last residues of her dream. She forced herself to think ahead to the end of her volunteer shift, to meeting up with Amy and Flory in the school cafeteria at lunch and making plans for Saturday.

This would be the May long weekend, the start of cottage season at Cultus Lake. The three best friends had been spending weekends and summers there for as long as they could remember, and Amy's parents still had their old cabin on the south shore. The girls would help the MacGillivrays air out the cabin and take the plastic off the furniture Saturday morning, and then Amy's mom would send them to Logan's Market for groceries for the first big feast of the season. It was tradition. There would be a dance Saturday night, and canoeing on Sunday, or maybe even swimming if this weather kept up. And then another whole day of it on Monday! Jane was eager to see which of the nests along the lakeshore would be filled with newly hatched robins and jays, all calling for food. Their cries started at first light, just after 4:00 a.m. She'd hear them long before she saw them.

A car horn blared up ahead, bringing her back to the present. Traffic had slowed on the curve leading round to Cedar's Ridge High. Jane geared down and went back to wondering what she'd wear to the dance on Saturday night. Flory would have something new, as usual, and it wouldn't matter what Amy wore—that girl would look great in a burlap sack. The cars sped up again, and Jane shifted into third. Maybe she'd have time for a trip to her favorite vintage shops tomorrow after school.

Rounding the corner in front of the school, dreaming of dresses and dancing, she almost missed it—a crow lay in the middle of the curb lane, small, and black, and still.

And alive, she knew.

Still alive.

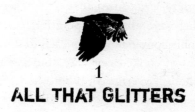

1
ALL THAT GLITTERS

J ANE REACHED into the dish with her tweezers and picked up one fat blueberry. Leaning forward, she held the blueberry above the small black head, just out of reach, and watched as bright, intelligent eyes followed her every move. Like a hypnotist, she began to move the blueberry through the air in slow, small circles, clockwise and then counterclockwise, watching for signs that her patient would soon respond. She opened her mouth, about to offer a few whispered words of encouragement, when her training kicked in and she closed it again, remaining silent. Patiently, she continued with her circles, until at last the fledgling crow opened its beak. Quickly, she dropped the plump morsel onto the sliver-thin pink tongue and sat back in her chair, grinning in satisfaction as the little bird gobbled like a tiny turkey. Try as she might, though, she couldn't convince him to take another berry.

Not hungry this morning, hey, Jane thought, as she reached down with the tweezers and plucked up another blueberry. *Well, your siblings look like they might appreciate my services!* Sure enough, the other two crows in the basket were already gaping for food, and Jane had no trouble convincing them each to down a berry, a tweezerful of cooked egg yolk, and a small chunk of raw salmon. *Dessert first? What was I thinking? Or maybe you three like that stinky fish best?* She smiled to herself and reached forward to tempt the first crow again with a juicy piece of salmon. But he held his beak resolutely shut.

Jane dropped the tweezers into the dish and grabbed a light towel from the top of the basket. Reaching in through the opening, she scooped the little crow from his perch and brought him to her lap, careful to keep his head and eyes covered so that he wouldn't be afraid. She made a mental note to find out later whether there was some state of matter that was solid, liquid, and gas all in one, because if there was, that's what a bird was. The crow felt like nothing in her hands—light, feathers, air—and at the same time like the pure essence of life itself, breathing, beating, warm blood, bones. She thought of the crow she had brought to the Center that morning, still struggling for life in the exam room. It, too, had felt this way in her hands. So vulnerable she could crush it if she chose to; so strong it could fly.

Or would be able to soon, if it recovered. Jane shuddered and shook her head, bringing her attention back to the animal in her hands. She flipped the little fledge onto his side and smoothed the feathers away from the keel bone that ran down the center of its breast. The skin there was taut, and the muscle mass surrounding the keel was firm. Despite the fact that he would not take food from her, this was not a malnourished or dehydrated bird. Righting him, Jane gently palpated the crop at the base of his throat with the tips of her thumb and forefinger. *There. Full of food. I knew it! You're eating on your own!*

Returning the crow to his perch, Jane moved to make a note on the case tag attached to the basket. If this bird was consistently self-feeding, there was no need to keep him on rounds. He would be moved to a larger aviary where he could learn to fly.

Suddenly, there was a rush of air, and black feathers blinded her. Jane cried out, lunging back and throwing her arms up to protect her face. The crow dropped to her chest and held fast to her sweatshirt with its toes, croaking and pecking, pulling at something near her throat.

"Bird out?" asked a wry voice behind her. Evie Jordan, the head of animal care at the Urban Wildlife Rescue Center (UWRC), reached around with an expert hand and pulled the eager little crow off of Jane. Jane dropped her arms then turned to face Evie, grateful for the help and still so relieved to have found her behaving like her usual self when she'd arrived this morning. She had taken Jane's rescued crow fledge and examined him right away, then commenced treating him for shock.

She had also reassured Jane that he was very likely to survive.

"Looks like this youngster spotted your feather pendant, Jane," Evie said now as she secured the three crows behind the basket's closure. "They're suckers for all that glitters."

Jane tucked the slender silver feather beneath her sweatshirt and looked sheepishly up at Evie. Her whole world had shrunk to the size of a basket with three fledgling crows inside, and as usual she'd tuned out every other sight and sound to concentrate solely on the animals in her care. She'd forgotten there was anyone or anything else around. Now, as the whole of the animal care room flooded back into focus, Jane noticed she was sitting in the middle of a three-ring circus.

It was 8:15 on Thursday morning, just before the start of the May long weekend, and baby bird season at the UWRC was well underway. The tables running along the perimeter of the care room were stacked two and three high with cages, kennels, and baskets—robins, crows, and jays—and the larger wooden aviaries in each corner, often empty through the winter, were now filled with chickadee, sparrow, and starling fledges all calling for food. The room's center table, which Jane was accustomed to using as a workspace, was laden with seven kennels: three gulls, two mallard ducks, and two mature starlings. On the floor, a large covered pen housed two more gulls, and at the far end of the room near the outside door, a pair of Canada geese occupied a second floor pen. Of the three thousand animals the UWRC took in throughout the year, two thousand of them would arrive between now and September. The air that swirled around her was warm and dense with noises and smells. Jane took a deep breath and grinned.

Down the hall, Jane could hear receptionist Anthony Lau fielding calls from the public about nests in their eaves, crows in their fruit trees, and lone birds on the ground that didn't seem to know how to fly. Isolation Room 1 had been outfitted with an incubator, and ice cream buckets had been turned into nests for altricial nestlings—those that hatched naked, blind, and unable to perch or stand or feed themselves. Ducklings and goslings—precocial babies—hatched covered in down, could see and walk or swim, and could feed themselves almost immediately. All of those at the Center right now were outside in heated brooders, likely peeping away in anticipation of their morning meal.

A timer rang, and Jane saw Beth Bozi rush from the kitchen back to ISO 1, a tray of small dishes in her hands. A university student hired by the UWRC to work full-time for the busy summer season, Beth had started feeding those nestlings at 7:00 that morning, and someone would feed them every fifteen minutes until dark. Through the window, Jane could see Frank Graves, the other summer staffer, hanging towels and sheets on the line outside. The drone of the washers and dryers down the hall would provide a non-stop soundtrack for the summer, Jane guessed, and the floor-to-ceiling shelves, normally bursting with neatly folded towels, stood almost empty.

Evie entered the care room again and collected a starling from the center table to be weighed and medicated in the examination room. Jane cleaned behind her, noting that the case tag on the starling's cage read "oiled." Had there been another oil spill? She reminded herself to ask when Evie returned.

Jane Ray had been volunteering with the Urban Wildlife Rescue Center since the previous October, when she'd rescued a surf scoter from drowning in Vancouver's Burrard Inlet after a canola oil spill. The work here was dirty, hard, and often heartbreaking. Her patients included the injured, the orphaned, and animals made sick by pollutants like oil, pesticides, and garbage. Many of the animals who made it to the Center did not make it back to the wild. Those who did survive and heal made the struggles and disappointments bearable. Jane had held many a bird in her own hands at that liminal moment when it ceased being captive and became wild again. Her shift earned her work experience credits at school, but she'd have done it anyway. She loved it.

The screen door slammed and Avis charged in carrying what appeared to be twice her own body weight in soiled towels. "Geese!" she exclaimed before retreating to the laundry room. Jane could have guessed by the smell. She remembered her first meeting with Avis Morton, a formidable older woman possessed of a sharp tongue that hid a remarkably kind heart. Jane had written her off immediately as a crotchety old bat, but had been surprised to discover a real friend concealed within the brusque, opinionated taskmaster. Tall and slim, her silver bob impeccable and her clothes incongruously stylish, Avis emerged from the laundry room completely untouched by her close encounter with the poopy towels. "Coffee at 11:00," she chimed, glancing up at the clock as another timer rang. "It'll likely be our last chance to take a break in the middle of a shift until September, so mind you're not late. And speaking of late, that's your timer, Jane Ray!" She zipped through the kitchen and out the screen door.

Last fall, Avis's rebuke would have soured her morning. Today, Jane grinned and called after her, "You mean it gets busier than this?" She could hear Avis cackling all the way down the path.

"What's so funny? Are you two laughing at me?" Katrina D'Angelo, another Thursday morning regular whom Jane knew from school, shuffled slowly through the care room carrying an armload of towels and a cardboard kennel. Sucking in her cheeks to hide her grin, Jane had to admit Katrina did look a bit the worse for wear. Her normally tanned and rosy complexion was haggard, and dark circles rimmed her eyes. Strands of honey-blond hair shot out at all angles from the rubber-band-secured bun on the top of her head.

"Tough track and field session yesterday?" Jane asked the athletic girl, trying to keep a straight face. It looked rather like she could have used a few more hours of sleep.

"More like a long post-track session with Mike," Katrina moaned, but with a wink. "Sometimes my own social schedule is too much, even for me!" Katrina made a grab for a second kennel on her way out the back door. "I'm off to clean the brooders," she threw back over her shoulder. "Avis won't touch them. Those ducklings had better behave, because I am *so* not in the mood!"

Jane's smile faded, and she hoped meanly that the ducklings would do their worst. Katrina D'Angelo was dating Mike MacGillivray, her best friend Amy's older brother and a boy she'd known all her life. Though she had no romantic designs on him herself, she had never understood what he saw in Katrina. Sure, she was tall, pretty, and athletic, but . . . oh, well, *duh*. She was only every grade twelve boy's dream date. Jane suspected that what was really bothering her was a confession Mike had made to her in secret the previous fall.

Ever since she could remember, Mike MacGillivray had been planning to attend university and study engineering. He'd spent his childhood preparing by taking apart Amy's toys and his mom's appliances and putting them back together again. Well, some of them, anyway.

Already, his proud parents were boasting to their friends about their engineer son. But after spending last summer working on an organic farm, Mike had decided he wanted something else. Strangest of all, he'd said it was Jane's fight against the oil company and her commitment to saving the animals that had convinced him to change his course. Problem was, he still hadn't told his parents of his decision, university applications were due this month, and Mike's high school graduation was only five weeks away. Jane was pretty sure he hadn't told Katrina his secret either. Heck, that girl probably thought GMO stood for Glamor Makeup Organizer. *Ooo, that's petty*, she thought.

"Jane, was that my timer or yours?" Beth interrupted Jane's thoughts as she sifted through the fresh laundry pile looking for small towels.

"Oh my gosh, Beth, that was mine!" Jane spun on her heel, grabbed the fledge timer and reset it for forty-five minutes. Turning back, she raced into the kitchen to start fresh diets. This round, she'd clean all the fledges' cages and feed them fresh food. Between rounds, she'd clean and feed the care room's regular patients, and if she had any time to spare, she'd start a couple loads of laundry. *And prep Katrina's duckling diets for her*, she thought to herself. *To make up for my nasty thoughts.*

The next time Jane glanced up at the clock, it read 11:03. Late for coffee. She was destined to be late all day, it seemed. Everybody cleaned and fed, except for two oiled starlings and three pigeons being treated for poisoning. She wanted to ask Evie about those. Laundry going. Duckling diets sitting on the kitchen counter waiting for Katrina. Jane checked her timer. She could take twelve minutes off before her fledges would be calling for food again.

Hurrying into the exam room to wash her hands, Jane caught sight of a small black form out of the corner of her eye. She turned to find the crow she'd rescued that morning lying lifeless on the admissions counter. Its head lay at a strange angle, stiff wings stood out slightly from the sides of its body, and around one thin black leg was tied a small square of manila cardboard. Jane felt her own body go cold. Slowly, her hand trembling, she reached for the small manila square, dreading what she might find. This was no ordinary case tag. Turning it over, she read the crude black letters in disbelief: **SAVE PEOPLE. KILL CROWS.**

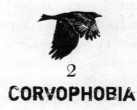

2
CORVOPHOBIA

JANE'S VISION BLURRED and she felt her body go limp. Just before she slumped to the floor, strong arms caught her and lifted her off the ground. The next thing she knew, she was seated in the receptionist's chair accepting a cup of cold water from Anthony and listening to a distant voice say, "Not your crow. Not your crow." She looked up into a haze of anxious faces as Evie, Avis, Beth, Frank, Katrina, and Anthony all crowded around the reception desk.

"What happened?" she whispered, her throat tight.

"The crow you saw in the exam room is *not* the one you rescued this morning, Jane." The voice belonged to Daniel Jackson, vet student, staff member, and Evie's second in command at the UWRC. He stood behind her now, his warm hands resting steadily on her shoulders, and Jane took in a deep, ragged breath and let it out again slowly. "Your crow is still resting on heat and seems to be stable. The crow you saw, the one that . . ." He paused. "Evie, maybe you want to handle this one?"

Evie nodded. "Right. Well, I was going to come and

talk to you all during your break, but I hadn't counted on Jane beating me to the punch." She gave Jane a rueful smile. "Someone is killing crows, and they want the UWRC to do the same." The Thursday morning crew looked uneasily around at one another, and without a word looked back at Evie, waiting for her explanation.

"What Jane just found in the exam room is the fourth crow delivered dead to the UWRC this week. I expect we'll find another on our doorstep early tomorrow morning." Evie spoke plainly and directly, but she paused here to clear her throat, and Jane understood that it was costing her a great deal to keep her emotions in check. "Each one had its neck broken, and each arrived with a threatening message tied to one leg." She stopped again, and Jane saw that her hands were shaking.

"Today's says, 'Save people. Kill crows,'" Jane finished for her.

There was a moment when the only sound in the small reception area was the hum of the computer on Anthony's desk. Then eight voices erupted at once.

"This is a crime!"

"Somebody should set a leg-hold trap tonight and see who gets caught in it!"

"Oh, don't be ridiculous."

"Do you know who did this?"

"Why would *anyone* do this?"

"Have you called the police?"

"Don't be *ridiculous!*"

"Never mind the police—we should get an attack dog!"

"*Ridiculous!*"

"A *rabid* attack dog!"

"Stop it," Evie said fiercely. "*Stop it!* There are injured animals recovering in the exam room. Keep your voices down." She looked suddenly weary and older than her twenty-five years. "We haven't decided yet how to respond. It has to be a joint decision of the UWRC board and staff, and our first consideration has to be the safety of the animals in our care."

Avis was the first to recover her senses. "Evie, what do you think is going on?"

Evie nodded at the longtime volunteer as if glad to hear at least one sensible question. "Avis, my honest answer is that I don't know. But my best guess is that it has something to do with West Nile Virus. We've been lucky in British Columbia so far: WNV has swept all the way across Canada and been held back by the Rocky Mountains. And it's crossed the United States from the east coast to the west, and somehow been stopped by the invisible border between Washington State and British Columbia. Nobody knows why. But everybody agrees on one thing: it's just a matter of time til the virus crosses one of those lines and hits us. And with the warm weather and the mosquitoes hatching, the news media are running story after story saying this is going to be the year. As a result, people are, quite frankly, freaking out."

Anthony nodded vigorously, a lock of his mod black shag falling across his face. "Understatement, girl! Half the calls we get these days are from people slapping at mosquitoes with one hand and talking on their cell phones with the other and wanting me to tell them if they're going to die," the reception staffer exclaimed dramatically. "I swear, I am going to start saying yes just to liven up my little old day!"

Evie laughed along with the rest of them, and Jane felt herself relax slightly. "Evie, if West Nile Virus is transmitted by mosquitoes," she asked, "what's anybody got against crows?"

"Mosquitoes are the vectors, the transmitters. Corvids are the indicator species," Evie replied. "In BC, that includes crows, ravens, and jays."

"So how come nobody's leaving dead ravens or jays at the door?" Katrina asked. "Like, I mean, logically . . ."

"Because people hate crows," Daniel interjected vehemently. "They're dark, they're dirty, they're ugly. There's too many of them. They steal other birds' eggs. They eat other birds' young. They eat road kill. They eat garbage." Daniel was spitting out his words. "In the past, they were known for eating the dead in battlefields. They were considered ill omens by the superstitious, and there are still a whole lot of superstitious people in these supposedly scientific times. People *hate* them."

"Thank you for that passionate summary, Daniel," Evie struggled to suppress a smile. She looked around at the group. "Daniel, you see, *loves* crows. They're intelligent, social, curious, and communicative. And they're actually very clean birds, and one of the more beautiful to watch in flight. They've been known to make great pets—not that we as wildlife rehabilitators would know anything about that!—and they have even been known to learn human speech. They make tools, a talent thought until recently to belong only to primates, and they can use them to perform various tasks. They even play, chasing one another or sliding down snow banks just for fun. And as Jane found out this morning, they love a little glamor!"

"Oooh! Dress me up and call me a crow!" Anthony exclaimed.

Evie gave him a playful slug on the arm. "You? A pest animal? Never!"

Jane registered Evie's last words and straightened in her chair. "'Pest animal!' I can't stand that term. It's a complete oxymoron!"

"Well, it's certainly a moronic way of looking at nature, I'll agree," Evie responded. "But there are a lot of people out there who think of any animal who builds a nest in *their* tree or *their* attic, or eats from *their* garden or garbage can is a pest. Never mind that they built their houses and planted their gardens in the middle of the animals' home, and razed half a rainforest to do it!" She sighed. "The irony is, the ones people call pests—rats, raccoons, coyotes, crows—are the ones who've adapted best of all to living with us."

Jane's timer went off inside the pocket of her sweat-shirt. "Coffee's over!" Avis said tersely, clearly relieved to end the conversation. "Jane, you have fledges to feed. I'll go turn off the coffee pot. Maybe next week."

"We will keep all of you posted on West Nile developments, if there are any, and how they affect the UWRC," Evie said as they all made to return to their various workstations. "And we'll also let you know what happens with the crows." Her voice got quieter, but lost none of its intensity: "We'll do everything we can to ensure neither situation puts you—or any other volunteer—in danger."

Jane was making her way down the hall toward the care room when she felt a hand on her shoulder. She turned to find Evie following her. "In all the drama, I forgot we had some good news as well." She held a sheaf of papers out toward Jane: "Your contract is ready to sign, and the hybrid car will be here by the last week of June." She paused. "I just hope that after this morning's fiasco you still want to work with us."

"Are you kidding?" Jane exclaimed, then clamped her hand over her mouth, remembering the animals. Last fall, when funding had come through for a dedicated mobile rescue team and vehicle for the summer months, Evie had offered Jane one of the jobs. She'd hardly been able to believe it at the time, but now here she was just weeks away from starting. "Sign me up! Oh, wait . . . fledges first, contract second."

Evie flashed her an approving smile. "I'll leave the paperwork on the front desk."

Jane completed her last round in silence, replaying the conversations and events of the morning in her head. A few minutes after noon, fledges fed and cleaned once more and left in the afternoon volunteer's capable hands, Jane signed her contract, said her goodbyes to the Thursday morning posse and headed out to her car. Despite the good news about her job, Jane was aware that she'd never been so relieved to leave the wildlife center behind and return to school.

3

FLORY DELIVERS A HISTORY LESSON

"I F I'M READING THIS CORRECTLY . . ." Flory paused dramatically and leaned forward in the rickety wooden chair, squinting at the computer screen and making notes in a black file folder, " . . . it's entirely possible that Alexander the Great died of West Nile Virus."

"Talk about ancient history!" Amy snorted, never even looking up from the collection of test tubes, pipettes, and vials of colored liquids arrayed in front of her. She poured a vile-looking, viscous yellow substance from one of the test tubes into a globe-bottomed beaker and smiled in satisfaction as a putrid gas rose up in reaction. "Al died, oh, about twenty-three hundred years ago, Flor. How could that possibly have anything to do with Jane's dead crows?"

Jane was staring into the bottom of a plastic tumbler at the dregs of her lemonade, where an errant mosquito was taking his last swim. The air was hot and still, and she felt a single drop of sweat leave her right temple and slide down the side of her face. Unconsciously, she turned her head and wiped it away on her shoulder. It was 3:30 on Thursday afternoon, and the three best friends had retreated to the Shack, their private hideaway at the side of the MacGillivray house, as soon as school had let out. Jane Ray, Amy MacGillivray, and Flory Morales had known each other literally all their lives—their parents had gone to school together, been witnesses at each other's weddings, bought homes near one another on Cedar's Ridge, raised their children together—and the three girls' friendship had lasted beyond the carefree play of their younger years to weather the hardships and heartaches of their teens. Jane had shoved away all thoughts of her early-morning dream, her rescue of the fledge, and Evie's revelations about the UWRC's slaughtered crows until the moment she could share them with her two most trusted friends.

Now, she glanced up at Flory's small form hunched over the computer, long, blue-black hair swinging forward to hide her face, and then turned to stare hard at Amy. "What did you say?"

Amy looked up from her experiment, alerted by something in Jane's voice, and pushed an errant lock of curly red hair out of her face with one gloved hand. "Dead crows? Ancient history? I . . . actually, I don't remember. What *did* I say?"

"Ancient history," Jane repeated slowly. "Alexander the Great died in . . ."

"June 10, 323 BCE, to be precise," Flory stated,

turning her chair to face the two other girls. "Plutarch—you know, the Greek historian—kept excellent notes."

"But I thought Alexander the Great was assassinated," Jane pressed. "Poisoned. I'm sure that's what we learned in history class."

Flory pulled her black file folder from the table behind her and opened it, poised to read. Jane caught Amy's eye-roll from across the room and looked down to hide her smile. Flory's favorite after-school hobby was research, the way other people's was shopping or street hockey. Born into a long line of lawyers and doctors, the petite Filipina girl came by it naturally, but it never failed to amaze her friends how seriously she took it. At home in her family's condo, she maintained four tall black filing cabinets filled with files, and she had talked about needing a new one by September. She was blessed with a near-photographic memory, and anything that didn't stick she could find in a matter of seconds in her records.

"Alexander the Great died in Babylon at the age of thirty-two following a two-week fever," Flory read from her notes. "Theories about the cause of his death have included poisoning, assassination,"—here Flory nodded at Jane as if to applaud her friend's recall—"and a number of infectious diseases. He was, um, indiscriminate in his affairs, shall we say. His symptoms as recorded by Plutarch included continuous fever, chills, excessive perspiration, muscle pain, progressive weakness, exhaustion, diminished ability to think, stupor, irrational vocal outbursts, and hallucinations."

"But how does that prove it's West Nile?" Amy asked as she squeezed clear fluid from an eyedropper into a bubbling mixture in a triangle-bottomed beaker. "I mean, that's how Mike acts pretty much every morning of his life." Jane guffawed, remembering sleepovers at Amy's and summer mornings at the Cultus cottages when Mike did in fact look as though he could have been suffering from stupor, diminished ability to think, and partial paralysis. "Minus the dying part, of course," Amy conceded. "Why couldn't it be just a bad case of the flu?"

Jane broke in: "More importantly, what about the fact that West Nile Virus didn't appear in North America until 1999, and that newspapers say the first recorded case ever was in Uganda in 1937? West Nile didn't even exist in Alexander's time! And like Amy said, Flor, what's all this got to do with my crows?"

"Patience, my friends," Flory replied with maddening calm. "Consider the evidence: as for poison, Alexander—I'll call him Alex for economy's sake—had a severe fever. My research shows that few poisons could cause such a fever, and even fewer were actually available in Alex's time. Next, none of the infectious diseases found in the populations of Babylon and the surrounding area was mentioned by any of the historians who wrote about Alexander's death. In addition, any such diseases would have been likely to cause casualties among his troops as well, but no casualties were recorded. The same goes for the flu, Ame—highly contagious, would have felled more than a few troops. Sorry, but no cigars for you."

Amy left her experiment to foment on its own and took a seat across from Jane at the large wooden table in the center of the room: "Okay, so I'm listening." Jane nodded, too, feeling a slight fluttering in her stomach. She had a hunch she might not like all that Flory had to say.

"Alex's death occurred in Babylon in late spring," Flory continued, laying her facts out before them carefully like jewels, sparkling with meaning. Babylon was located on the Euphrates River and bordered on the east by a swamp, where birds and animals were plentiful and insects such as mosquitoes were also likely present." Jane glanced down into her lemonade and saw that the mosquito in the tumbler no longer moved. "The symptoms, the length of illness, and the environmental circumstances add up," Flory summarized. "But it is only the recent global emergence of the virus, coupled with a rereading of Plutarch's chronicles, that has led to the theory about West Nile." Flory looked up from her notes, her face alight with a triumphant grin.

"Uh, Flor, is there some sort of informational Bermuda Triangle in here? Because I did not understand whatever you did not just say," Amy said, running both gloved hands through her unruly mass of red curls until her hair stood out in all directions.

Jane nodded. "I have to admit I'm with Ame this time, Flor. And I still don't understand what any of this has to do with my crows!"

Flory lifted the top sheet of lined yellow paper from her file folder. Even in the dim light of the old gardening shed, Jane could see that it was entirely covered in her friend's tiny cursive. Flory read without looking up from the page: "Scientists studying West Nile have become aware that massive die-offs of corvids, the birds most susceptible to the virus, occur two to six weeks before an increased incidence of human illness. Crows and ravens especially are considered to be early-warning signals by officials. In Alexander's time, bird observers, or oracles, used the behavior of certain birds to predict the future. Whether or not Plutarch was such an oracle, he did describe Alexander's entrance into Babylon in this way, and I quote: 'When he arrived before the walls of the city he saw a large number of ravens flying about and pecking one another, and some of them fell dead in front of him.'" Flory lowered the sheet of paper to her lap and looked up, blinking. "A couple weeks later, Alex was dead." *

---

* I am quoting from Marr, J.S., and Calisher, C.H. Alexander the Great and West Nile virus encephalitis. Emerg Infect Dis: December 2003. Check out www.cdc.gov/ncidod/EID/vol9no12/03-0288.htm —F.M.

There was a moment of silence in the Shack as the three girls stared at one another. Then Jane's jaw dropped as something large and bubbly and greenish-yellow mushroomed up behind Amy's head. Jane's expression, coupled with an ominous gurgling sound, caused Amy to spin around just as her forgotten experiment erupted over the lab table in a mass of chartreuse foam and sulfurous stink. At that moment, Jane heard the creak of rusty hinges at her feet. Flory leapt onto her chair, screaming, and Jane looked down in time to see the trap door in the floor of the Shack rise slowly up from the ground.

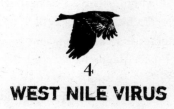

4

WEST NILE VIRUS

A LOUD BARK SOUNDED from the underground tunnel that ran between the Shack and the MacGillivray house, and a moment later, two heads emerged from the trap door: one sported a neat auburn coif and the other a shaggy mop of golden waves. Flory clapped a hand to her mouth as she recognized Mrs. MacGillivray and Buster, the family dog. Jane started to giggle. Amy began to holler as Buster scrambled up the last of the underground stairs and tore across the room, tail wagging furiously as he leapt up to give his mistress a sloppy wet kiss.

"Back off, Buster Brown, this place is practically a bio-hazard! Down, boy! Put that tongue back in your head, I'm telling you!" Amy dodged and danced, her gloved hands waving madly about as she tried to keep the eager retriever from touching any part of her latest disaster. "I can't believe I'm going to have to start this whole experiment all over again tomorrow. Buster, drop that! Dirty! Ten years, and he still thinks I'm secretly making food in here that I won't share with him. Good boy."

Mrs. MacGillivray's disembodied head let out a groan from the floor. "Why, oh, why couldn't I have had a *girl* for a daughter instead of a scientist? And what is that *smell*?" Buster padded over and licked her face in sympathy.

At this, Amy dropped her arms to her sides, sprouted a Botox-style pout and ambled, hips first, into the center of the small room. Jane and Flory whistled and made the appropriate catcalls. At five foot nothing, with generous curves, prominent features, and a mane of independent-minded red curls, Amy Airlie MacGillivray was not built for the catwalk. That said, she knew how to put on a show. She spun in place now, flashing the jeans and stained hoody she wore beneath her dad's old white work shirt, and then struck a provocative pose: "You got lucky, Mama MacGillivray," she intoned in a breathy voice. "You got both!"

At this, Flory fell off her chair laughing and Jane stared at her friend in wonder. A comment like that from her own mom would have left Jane fuming. But Amy somehow just turned it around and made it all better. And funny, too. How?

"God gave me crazy children, is what I got," Mrs. MacGillivray retorted, trying with limited success to keep her face straight. "One tries to blow up the house daily, and the other suddenly spends all his money on clothes and hair gel and smelly stuff he never bothered with before that girl. Now, I ask you!"

Jane's eyes widened, and Amy nodded. "Oh, yeah. Mike's gone all metrosexual lately, thanks to Ms. Katrina D'Angelo! Dressing up for school and reeking of cologne. Next thing you know, it'll be mani-pedicures and a chest wax. I mean, can you *imagine*? A MacGillivray man with no body hair? It's just wrong!"

Before Jane had a chance to answer, there was a sharp knock on the door of the Shack and two boys stepped inside. Benoît Tremblay took in Amy's pouty pose and made a beeline for her lips with his own. Mrs. MacGillivray cleared her throat loudly from the hole in the floor and Ben released his hold on the little redhead, startled. "Oh, allô, Mrs. Mac. I did not see you down there!" Stocky and dark, Ben was built like a Tasmanian devil—all shoulders and chest, and plenty of body hair. He'd entered grade twelve at Cedar's Ridge High half way through the year, and was doing well despite English being his second language. He'd arrived alone from a francophone community outside of Toronto, Ontario, wanting to spend some time on the west coast before graduating, and had found a one-woman welcome committee in Amy MacGillivray. Mark Co, Flory's boyfriend of three years, entered the Shack quietly behind Ben and crossed over to Flory, taking her outstretched hand.

"Perfect timing, boys!" the MacGillivray head exclaimed. "I was just about to ask these girls to clean up the yard for me and bring the groceries in from the car.

Many hands make light work! And Buster could use a little exercise while you're at it. Oh, and of course you're all welcome to stay for dinner. Veggie tortière and a salad, and fruit crèpes for dessert, specially for Ben." The trap door slammed shut and she was gone, her muffled footsteps disappearing down the underground corridor.

The three-storey MacGillivray home was an historic farmhouse, white with green shutters, that had sat on the north shore of Elfin Lake for almost a hundred years. To the east and west stretched acres of untouched woods—poplars, birches, cedars, and pine, and salmonberry bushes and brush that would provide summer cover to sparrows, black-capped chickadees, thrushes, and goldfinches. At the back of the house, to the north, a creek ran through the property and down to the lake, and an old access road led away from the woods back into the city. To the south lay Elfin Lake, and above it, Cedar's Ridge. The waters of the small lake, still in the afternoon heat, shimmered silver like a mirror beneath the glare of the sun. Jane watched paddleboats and canoes skim its surface and then let her gaze fall on her own home on the far side, a dark brown two-storey surrounded by towering cedars, its small boat dock jutting into the waters of the south shore. It would be empty right now. It would be empty, probably, until midnight. Dinner with the MacGillivray clan sounded like a good plan.

Flory and Mark took turns tossing a saliva-soaked throw-toy for Buster, and Amy and Ben began bagging the beech, maple, cherry, and birch branches that lay strewn across the expansive yard where Mr. MacGillivray had been pruning trees. They stopped every few feet to celebrate their accomplishments with a kiss. Amy had mentioned to Jane and Flory that Ben was teaching her francophone kissing. Like French only longer, she'd explained. She was clearly a keen student. Jane grabbed a garbage sack and pitched in. They'd never finish the job at this rate.

Eventually, Buster tired and stretched himself out on the lawn to chew his toy, and the five friends settled into a rhythm of collecting, bundling, and bagging branches. The conversation turned once again to the morning's mystery. Just as Amy and Flory had been, the boys were horrified to hear of the dead crows with the tags tied to their legs.

"And how is it that you do not yet have the West Nile here?" Ben asked, stunned. "It is everywhere in Canada, I was thinking. And almost everywhere in the United States, also!"

"It hasn't made it over the Rocky Mountains yet from the east," Jane answered, "and for some unknown reason it hasn't crossed the border from the south. Nobody knows . . ." Suddenly Jane gasped. "Hey, wait! You're from Ontario—you've seen it! What's it like?"

Ben grimaced. "It is craziness, Jane! You must

remember, you see, we had the SARS, where the people were afraid to leave their houses, or to go to the hospital if they were sick, or hug their friends. On the subway, everyone was wearing the masks, reading the newspaper for the day's terrible stories." Jane and the others nodded, remembering how some of those stories had made their way to Vancouver newspapers. "And there was the mad cow," Ben continued, "and foot-and-mouth disease and the . . . how do you say? Bio-terror, yes? With the anthrax. And of course 9-11 and the tsunamis and the hurricanes and the war. And now, the, the bird influence?"

"Influenza," Jane nodded, encouraging him to go on. "The avian flu."

"Yes. Avian flu," Ben repeated thoughtfully. "And all the time, the newspapers and the televisions and the radios and the Internet all have the giant headlines and the terrible stories and the predictions about so many things. So many things that never happened! But still everyone is listening and reading, at home, in the car, at work, at the pub. And now, everyone is terrified!"

Jane could picture it. She'd read it all herself in the local papers when West Nile hit Canada's east coast. The record sales of mosquito repellent, the pesticide spraying and the chemicals in lakes and marshes and ponds to kill the larvae, the lakeside cottages left empty all summer, owners too afraid to leave their concrete jungle for the real thing. Even people wearing clothing made of mosquito netting. Ben was right, it was crazy. But people went crazy when they got scared.

"But it's kind of like getting the flu, isn't it? West Nile, I mean?" Amy asked. "Most people don't even know they have it!"

At this, Flory dropped Buster's ball and ran toward the Shack. All activity ceased and the little group waited in silence until she returned, black file folder in hand.

"Most people who get it will never even know it," Flory confirmed, huffing a little from her run. She opened her file: "About twenty percent will experience mild symptoms that last less than a week. Less than one percent will get the severe form of the illness, and most of these will be people whose immune systems are already compromised, or who are over the age of fifty. That's the good news. The bad news is that, of those, five to fifteen percent will die."

"So, what exactly is 'mild?'" Amy inquired, crouching to resume tying a bundle of branches. Jane made a mental note to remind Mr. MacGillivray to do his pruning earlier next year. There could have been nests in these trees.

Flory read from her notes: "Fever, headache, muscle aches and pains, swollen lymph nodes . . ."

"So basically the flu," Amy interrupted, tying a slipknot and compressing the bundle.

" . . . and occasionally a skin rash on the trunk of the body," Flory finished.

Amy humphed, scratching absently at her torso.

"And severe?" Jane asked quietly, holding a bag open as Amy filled it with bundles of branches.

"Fever and headache again," Flory read, "neck stiffness, muscle weakness, stupor and disorientation, coma, and then death." She paused. "That's what it looks like from the outside. On the inside, either the brain itself, or the lining of the brain and spinal cord are swelling with encephalitis or meningitis, and there's no specific medication designed to treat it. Either the swelling stops, or it doesn't. If it does—if you recover, I mean—you're immune from West Nile Virus for life."

Jane wiped the sweat from her forehead, a thought suddenly occurring to her: "And is that how it goes in animals, too?"

Flory shook her head and flipped over the page. "Different symptoms, same cause. I'm sure the staff at the UWRC could tell you more, Jane, but my research indicates you'll see depression, anorexia or loss of appetite, green urates and diarrhea, uncoordinated body movements, severe tremors, seizures, and sudden death."

Jane frowned. "But those all sound like symptoms of CNS—central nervous system damage," she mused. "We get birds at the Center all the time who've flown into windows and present exactly like that. How will we be able to tell the difference?"

"You won't," Flory replied. "Except your West Nile

bird will likely be dead within 24 hours."

"And then your necropsy at the lab will tell you," Amy finished. Amy had applied for a summer job as a student intern at the provincial laboratories and was clearly anticipating the kind of task she might be faced with in the coming weeks.

Ben had grabbed a tennis ball from a bin at the side of the house, and he tossed it roughly to Mark. It made a sharp "thok!" as Mark caught it and tipped Jane's senses back into the present—the uncharacteristic heat of the May afternoon, the thousand spring greens of grass and rushes and leaves and hills, the hum of insects in Mrs. MacGillivray's flower beds, the soft smells of lake water and geraniums, fresh-cut grass, and her own sweat hanging warm in the air. She was mildly surprised at her ability to distinguish even those scents and knew that any other animal could identify a hundred more. Its life depended on it. She wondered what fear smelled like to an animal. And what did the city smell like, when all of its inhabitants suddenly went insane with fear? A ragged call pulled her gaze skyward, where six crows were making their way across the lake toward the northwest. As they passed over the poplars lining Elfin's north shore, they flushed another chorus of crows from the trees' branches, and then another, and another, and the growing gathering flew steadily northward until it passed behind a stand of cedars and out of sight.

"It's just crows that get it, though, right?" Amy asked,

winding twist ties around the tops of the garbage bags to close them. "Sorry, Jane, that came out wrong, no disrespect to crows. I meant, crows are the only animals that die from West Nile, right?"

"Crows. Ravens. Magpies. Jays." With each sharp word, Ben threw the ball with greater force. Mark suddenly had to work hard to keep up. Jane was surprised; she'd thought the boys had stopped listening. "Gulls. Cuckoos. Robins," Ben continued. "Eagles. Hawks. Kestrels. Kingfishers. Cranes. Cormorants. Pheasants. Flamingos. Herons. Mallards." Pausing with the ball in his hand, he glanced at Buster, and then over at Amy. "People's dogs. People's cats. My horse," he added quietly. "Many, many horses." He threw the ball hard and it went wide. Mark turned and ran down the lawn after it.

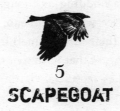

5
SCAPEGOAT

A MY MOVED TO STAND NEXT TO BEN, and they both stared out at the lake, not speaking. Flory cleared her throat. "Over a hundred and fifty species," she said, putting a number to Ben's frightening list. "But Amy is partly right, too. Ninety percent of all bird deaths occur in the corvid family. And what Ben said about horses . . ." She paused, looking at Ben's and Amy's backs. "It's bad. Of those infected by West Nile, about forty percent die."

"So let me get this straight," Jane said. This sultry, sweaty afternoon wasn't improving her mood the way she'd hoped, and neither was what she was hearing. "Mosquitoes give West Nile virus to humans, crows are victims, too, but somebody in Cedar's Ridge is killing crows and asking the wildlife center to do the same? I don't get it!"

Ben finally turned back and faced the little group. "What I am thinking is that the crow is just a goat."

Jane let out a nervous laugh but choked it back when she caught a stormy look from Amy. "Uh, what's that, Ben?"

But Flory was nodding as though Ben had made perfect sense. "I see what you mean, Ben, yes! People need a target for their fears, something to appease the angry forces of nature that have sent this disease down from the heavens. A sacrificial victim. And what better than a . . ."

"Scapegoat!" Jane smacked her palm to her forehead. "Of course! And since dead crows at New York's Bronx Zoo in 1999 were the first image North Americans had of West Nile Virus . . ."

"Yes, Jane! Flory exclaimed. "That's it! What people see is that first crows get sick, then people get sick. As if the crows caused it. But in fact, the crows are just the messengers."

"And now people are killing the messenger," Jane finished.

"Never mind that they're a bizillion times more likely to die of obesity-related diseases than West Nile Virus," Amy muttered, still sullen. The conversation had put the whole company into a foul mood, Jane noticed, and not even the warmth of the sun could burn off the tense chill. She wished she could think of a way to change the subject, but the conversation was rolling at full speed and she couldn't find the brakes.

Mark, usually silent and always thoughtful, spoke now. "If those 1999 crows didn't bring West Nile Virus to North America, then how *did* it get here?" He peered over Flory's shoulder at the contents of her black file folder as if searching for an answer.

"There are a number of theories," she replied, nestling back against him. "It could have been brought over by migratory birds that were already infected. A local mosquito takes a blood meal from one of them on this end, another meal from a local bird, and *voilà*, the transmission has begun. Or a person with the virus could have arrived on an international flight. A mosquito bites her and then bites a bird. Another theory revolves around the importing—legal or illegal—of birds from a country where West Nile was already prevalent. And of course virus-carrying mosquitoes themselves could have hitched a ride on a New York-bound aircraft. Any one of these ... Jane? What is it?"

A fifth possibility had entered Jane's mind, one that frightened her in a way the four others did not, one she would have preferred not to say out loud. But it was too late. Her face had given her away. Her mind had pulled disparate ideas and images from the afternoon's conversations—Alexander the Great dying in Babylon, Flory's infected mosquitoes hitching rides on New York-bound airplanes, Ben's talk of 9/11 and the anthrax scare.

"Flory," Jane said carefully, "where is Babylon?"

Flory shut her black file folder, eyes wide. "Babylon? It doesn't exist any more, Jane. Why? I mean, it's not called that any more. Babylon was the capital city of Mesopotamia. Now, the country is called Iraq, and the capital city is Baghdad ... Oh! Oh, Jane, you're not thinking . . . ?" Flory was starting to put the pieces together the same way Jane had done.

"I don't know," Jane answered, even more frightened now that Flory had recognized the same possibility.

"Don't know *WHAT*?" Amy yelled in frustration.

"Whether West Nile Virus was introduced to North America as an act of bioterrorism," Mark said softly, having followed the girls' thinking.

"Or whether governments would merely like us to think so in order to justify a war," Flory interjected darkly.

Ben, suddenly pale despite the heat and hard work, looked miserable. "You see? *You see?* Already you are going crazy, and it has not yet even arrived!"

"Ben's right," Amy snapped, her Scottish practicality rising suddenly to the surface. "That *is* crazy. Who's for a game of touch football?"

Ben couldn't help smiling and crossed the yard to grab Amy in a mock tackle. Jane felt like doing the same. Her pragmatic friend had finally cut the tension of the afternoon, and the relief in the little group was palpable. Buster must have sensed it, too. He trotted over to Ben and dropped his ball in front of the boy, ready for more games.

"Less work, more play, right, boy?" Amy said, fondling the top of the scruffy blond head. Jane thought, not for the first time, about how animals understood the concept of balance a whole lot better than people.

She'd spent her entire day, it seemed, trying to shake off a dark mood, and Buster had got it in one. "Guys, you up to the challenge?" Amy tossed the ball high into the air, face-off style. "Girls, let's get tonight's dinner out of the back of the Love-Mobile."

Jane, Amy, and Flory headed for the garage and the MacGillivray's ancient brown station wagon. As they passed a birdbath suspended from the branches of an old pear tree, Flory stopped to deliver a brief lecture: "Amy, you will want to remind your parents to remove all standing water from the yard in anticipation of mosquito season. There's no sense in taking any unnecessary risks or endangering . . . hey!"

Amy winked at Jane over Flory's head. Jane had seventeen years of interpreting those winks. Without hesitating, she stepped behind Flory and pinned her arms. In a single motion, Amy lifted the basin out of its chain-link hanger and drenched the poor girl from shoulders to toes in slimy green birdbath. Screaming now, Flory beelined to the garden hose that lay coiled against the side of the house, cranked open the faucet and turned it, full blast, on her two friends. Jane stood in the cold spray, laughing.

Amy ducked into the garage and returned holding a bag of groceries up in front of her like a shield. She grabbed something from inside the bag and threw it at Flory. Reflexively, Flory turned, and the ripe tomato splatted like a paintball bullet all over the back of her white T-shirt. Spinning around, the hose still spraying water at full force, Flory aimed the nozzle at Amy and her bag of edible armor. The brown paper bag quickly gave way, and three more tomatoes plopped onto the grass. While Amy struggled to salvage the remaining groceries, Jane and Flory ran forward, scooped up the tomatoes and pelted each other. "Amy, there's a mosquito on your forehead!" Jane screamed. "I'd better get that for you!" She beaned the beleaguered red-head with an especially soft tomato. As more groceries fell to the ground, Jane and Flory retrieved them and bombarded Amy from both sides.

From down by the lake, there was a sudden yell, and then a splash. One of the boys had thrown the ball too far and Buster had happily leapt into the lake after it. Jane glanced back in time to see the soaked and ecstatic dog tearing up the lawn toward the girls, fur streaming, Ben and Mark calling to him futilely and struggling to catch up. "Back off!" she yelled to Flory as Buster took air for the last couple of yards. He landed squarely on top of Amy, paused to give himself a thorough shake, then bent forward to lick tomato juice from his mistress's face.

The two boys came to a full stop at the sight of the girls and stared, open-mouthed. "Is chivalry dead?" Amy moaned pitifully from under the dog. She sat up slowly as if wounded in battle. Then reaching behind her quickly with both hands, she grabbed the closest pieces of produce and flung them at the boys. The strawberries found their marks with satisfying splats. Jane and Flory bent double, laughing so hard they were crying.

"Yoohoo, kids . . . dinner is . . . !"

Mrs. MacGillivray's suspended call hung in the air like a guillotine blade. All heads whipped around to face the front deck, where the MacGillivray matriarch stood, hands on her hips, eyes blazing. In the silence, Jane heard the distant shouts of happy canoers on the water. *Oh, to be far, far out on the lake at this moment,* she thought.

"What . . . in THUNDER . . . have you people DONE . . . with *MY DINNER*?" Mrs. MacGillivray's face was alight with a fury only the Scottish can muster outside of wartime.

Flory crossed herself reflexively, and as she glanced around, noticed with horror they were all on the verge of looking like entrants in a wet T-shirt contest.

"I think we're going to have to go to the cleaner's," Amy muttered without shifting her gaze from her mother or moving her lips.

"Uh, I think we're going to have to go to the grocery store first," Jane replied in the same way.

Flory raised her eyes skyward: "I think I'm going to have to go to Confession."

6
CEDARS MEDITERRANEAN CAFÉ

I T WAS DARK by the time Jane dropped Flory off at
home. A perfect half moon lit a few small clouds
in the eastern sky, and stars winked and shone above
in patterns Jane wished she knew. What would it be
like to go through school all over again, she wondered,
now that I know what I'd listen for, now that I know
what matters to me? Not battle dates or parentheti-
cal clauses or popularity contests. But the names of
things—flowers, trees, the constellations. How a hum-
mingbird finds its way from South America to Alaska
and back every year. How a star can send its insistent
message of light to the earth, long light years after it has
faded to black.

Dinner had started late—after groceries had been
replaced and stained clothing set to soak in the basement
sink—and threatened to be a tense affair, until the three
girls and the two boys had appeared in the kitchen in
various combinations of ancient MacGillivray gardening grubbies. Try as she might to stay angry, Amy's
mom couldn't help but laugh at the motley group. Over

a meal made more delicious by the late hour and their time spent outdoors, Amy's parents and the five friends had left the day's worries behind and talked only of their plans for the upcoming long weekend at Cultus Lake.

"So we'll go straight from school tomorrow?" Flory called back now as she headed up the front steps of the Moraleses' townhouse.

Jane nodded and waved through the open window. "I'll pick you up in the morning and we can just leave our stuff in the trunk for the day. 'Night, Flor!" She put the car into gear and headed east across the ridge, letting the cooling breeze play across her face and through her hair. It was a relief after the day's relentless heat. Turning down the long, steep drive that led to the Ray home, she remembered a moment before it appeared below her that the house would be dark. Earthen-brown against obsidian forest against steel lake. Not even a porch light. It was Jane's job to make sure the house looked lived-in in the evenings, while her mom and dad were at the restaurant. She'd forgotten. Well, she'd had a very dramatic day. Although she somehow doubted that would wash with her mom if the house had been robbed.

The cats greeted her at the basement door, Sweet Pea rubbing against her ankles as Minnie flopped on top of her feet. "Alone all this time in the dark, and you're not even mad at me!" Jane said, scooping Minnie up for a full-body hug. "Well, that'll change when you realize

I'm going out again!" Jane climbed the stairs and strode from room to room, turning on lights and checking for evidence of criminal activity. Nothing. Burglars would have taken one look at the Rays' shabby old stuff and headed for greener pastures. "Good guard kitties!" Jane teased, turning to stroke the soft little forms that followed closely at her heels. In the kitchen, she topped up their food and water and set out two small dishes of treats. As she sat on the back of the couch listening to the comforting crunching sounds they made, she wished she could just pull on her pyjamas, crawl into bed, and wait for the two of them to hop on top of her for the night. "In a couple of hours, I promise," she said. "I haven't seen them all week, and if I don't go tonight, I might not see them til next Tuesday." Before she could change her mind, she slipped down the stairs again and was gone.

Cedars Mediterranean Café was less than a mile from home, on High Street, in the short block of restaurants and stores that lay between the civic square and Shopping City Mall. Jane zipped down the back alley, pulled into the tiny lot, and swung open the heavy back door. Alley, cars, and dumpsters disappeared, and she was in another world.

Garlic and olive oil, cinnamon and warm honey. Heat, waves of it suspended in the air—the ovens, the stove, the grill, the rotisserie. The dishwasher's whish and hum. The clink and bustle of glasses, dishes, cutlery, roasting pans, pastry sheets. Snippets of songs her grandmother had sung her, competing songs on the stereo, shouts and the laughter of guests, the familiar rhythms of her dad's voice as he called instructions to his sous-chef, Marcello. Kitchen to the left, office and washrooms to the right. And straight ahead, in the dining room, there was Effie, arms straining with laden plates, smiling and flushed, and Elias, her husband, clearing tables and serving drinks, turning down the lights and turning up the music.

Jane stepped into the kitchen and pulled a stool over to the island in the center of the room. Her dad turned from the far counter, a diamond-shaped piece of *baklava* in one hand and a dish of figs and yogurt in the other, and set them down in front of her. He'd known she was there. She grinned up at him. "I can't sit long," he said, pulling up a second stool. "Learn anything fun today?"

Marcello leaned in from the oven to add slices of honey-baked pear to her dish. Jane caught herself staring at the dark curls escaping from beneath his chef's hat and blushed. The tall Italian was a recent graduate of the local culinary academy, winning her dad over by mastering the Ray family recipes and charming everyone else in the restaurant with guileless self-confidence. He gave Jane a huge, bright-eyed smile before turning back to his work. Jane blushed, noticed with relief that everyone else in the kitchen was rosy with the heat, and hoped she hadn't revealed her crush. *Way too old for me*, she reminded herself, shaking her head.

Between bites of pastry and fruit, Jane told her dad about her early-morning rescue, the looming threat of West Nile Virus, the dead crows delivered to the UWRC, and the conversations at the MacGillivrays'. "I can't imagine school is nearly so exciting," he teased her, breaking off a piece of *baklava* for himself.

She laughed. "But what do you think, dad?" she asked him. "Would somebody really . . . ?"

"Joe, there's somebody out front wants to know whether you'll honor a coupon from another restaurant. Oh, hi Jane! Effie can't talk sense into them. Maybe you can. I mean, we start giving out random discounts and turning this place into Family McJoint, and there goes all my hard work!" Jane's mom had started talking as she left the office down the hall, paused briefly in the kitchen doorway to blow her husband a kiss, and then continued on her way toward the dining room, talking all the while.

"Right there, Ellen," Jane's dad called after her, as he stood to wash his hands. He winked at Jane—"They call that the Doppler effect, right?"—and hurried out of the kitchen.

Jane half smiled. She often thought of her dad as a human being and her mom as a human doing, almost a cartoon character in the way she sped from office to kitchen to dining room to bar, never still for longer than a frame or two, visible only as a trail of color leading off the edge of Jane's vision. Her dad was right—she could almost hear the sound effects.

This was the way things were now—two parents, three jobs, more money, no time. Nobody ever home but the cats. Her dad had opened Cedars just over four years ago, and the investment had put the family in dire financial trouble. They'd almost lost their home on Elfin Lake, had had to sell their camper van and their cottage at Cultus, and their contented family of three had become a tense duo, Jane and her mom, as her dad had practically moved into the restaurant in a superhuman effort to keep the struggling business afloat.

Just before the end of last year, Jane had exploded on her mom, letting out four years of frustration and hurt in one long stream, and accusing her of standing by and watching as her dad failed. Ellen Ray had fired back, telling her, essentially, to grow up. Things change. Their family had changed. But she also acknowledged that she had never offered to help Joe, too angered by loss and loneliness to feel like a partner in his grand venture. The argument had surprised them, and hurt them both, but each had taken the other's words to heart. For Ellen's part, she had shouldered the marketing and promotion of the restaurant, eking out scraps of time in the early mornings and late at night so as not to affect her full-time job as promotions director for a Yaletown public relations firm. That job was the Ray family's lifeline, and she couldn't let it go until the restaurant was turning a healthy profit. She called on all her skills—and pulled in a few favors—to get restaurant reviews in all the papers, sponsor wine-tastings with chic labels, and host special events for leading business people in the community. Between her efforts and Joe's way of remembering his customers' names and favorite dishes, Cedars was finally taking off. They'd had to hire more staff, reservations were a must for dinner, and everyone in the city, it seemed, was trying to get a table for Saturday nights.

Jane had gotten what she wanted—and a whole lot of other things she'd never imagined. Her dad was more busy, not less. Her mom never came straight home from work any more, and despite Jane's love for Sweet Pea and Minnie, the house always felt empty. Worst of all, Joe and Ellen seemed to be on their second honeymoon, smooching in the back hallway of the restaurant so often they could probably teach Amy and Ben a few things. It was disgusting. What had she done? The family had changed again, and this time she couldn't complain. She'd gotten what she wanted. The problem was, she just didn't know where in this new family she belonged.

A sudden rush of street sounds and car horns told

her the front door had opened. Jane stood up from the island and stepped into the hallway to check out the new arrivals. Lightening fast, she backed up into the kitchen again, heart racing, almost knocking a platter of food out of the sous-chef's hands.

"Oh, Marcello, I'm so sorry!" She forgot to blush, she was so startled by what she'd seen. She heard Effie greet the newcomers as though they were regulars, asking if they wanted their usual table. Slowly, she peered around the corner again. Yes, she'd been right. There in the back booth, holding court with three of his cronies and laughing loudly enough to drown out every other sound in the restaurant, was Cedar's Ridge City Councilor Rand Harbinsale.

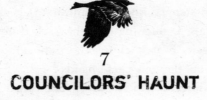

7

COUNCILORS' HAUNT

"I SHOULD HAVE TOLD YOU," Jane's dad said apologetically, as she leaned heavily against the island, breathing hard. "They've been coming in every Thursday night for the past couple of months. Whenever it came to mind, you weren't around." His frown deepened. "Or I guess I should say, I wasn't around. When you came in tonight, I just didn't think of it."

Salt-and-pepper-haired, movie-star handsome, and aggressively charismatic, Randall Harbinsale was a member of Cedar's Ridge City Council and General Manager of the Cedar's Ridge Golf & Country Club. He was also the father of Jane's ex-boyfriend, Jake.

It doesn't matter, Jane wanted to say. *It was December when he broke it off. I'm* way *over it.* But the sight of Jake's dad—a bigger, older, more confident version of the boy who'd asked her out last fall, who'd championed her fight against SeaKing Shipping, who'd kissed her for the first time—called all those memories back with an intensity that brought surprise tears to her eyes. Rand Harbinsale had not been fond of her. She'd always wondered whether he had something to do with his son's decision to stop seeing her. Jake had ended it so suddenly, when everything was going so well, and in such a cowardly way. He'd never sought her out to explain; in fact, she couldn't recall seeing him since. She'd heard weird rumors—that he'd eloped with Leila Collins, that he'd been offered a basketball scholarship by an American college. She'd ignored them, and everything to do with him, until she could say his name without choking up. It had taken a couple of months. And now here she was practically crying. Unconsciously, she put her hand to her heart.

Marcello had made her a latté, extra milk, and he set it down on the island with a flourish. "Decaf, Marcello?" she asked. "I need my beauty sleep, you know." She ventured a wan smile.

"You need none of the beauty aids, Miss Ray," Marcello replied, bowing. "But yes, it is of course decaf." He turned back to the vegetables on the grill, smiling broadly. *A girl could forget what she was sad about with compliments like that*, Jane thought. *Too old*, she reminded herself, *way too old*.

"Who are the others, dad?" she asked as she sipped the rich beverage. It felt good in her hands, despite the heat of the kitchen. "With Mr. Harbinsale, I mean."

"All city councilors," he answered, his back to her as he seasoned a plate of sliced eggplants. "The woman is Margaret Moody—Madge, they call her. Just Plain

Moody, according to your mother. Can't see it myself, really. She seems like somebody's sweet little auntie, those sausage curls and the flowered dresses and cardigans. Very knowledgeable about plants. Gets me all my herbs."

Jane smiled. Her dad had a way of seeing the best in everyone, even when there wasn't much best to see. Her mom, on the other hand . . . Jane found her own version of the truth often lay somewhere between their two opinions. "Madge Moody," she pondered aloud. "Her name sounds familiar for some reason."

"Gardening column in the local paper," her dad answered. "And she owns Cedar's Ridge EarthWorks garden shop. Miraculous green thumb, by all accounts."

"And the tall, lopey blond guy?"

"Gordon Gunnarson. Goes by 'Buzz,'" her dad chuckled, lining a casserole dish with the eggplant. "Could be because he's a barber. Or it could be all the developments he's approved." Joe Ray mimicked chain-sawing through his chopping block. "Of course, Elias's theory is that he's always a bit buzzed. Elias would know—he serves the drinks!" Joe laughed. "Harmless fellow if you ask me. Bit of a fence sitter in council, I hear, waits to see which way the wind's blowing before he'll vote. The city's seen worse."

Jane couldn't see a man like Rand Harbinsale cozying up to someone such as her dad had just described.

Maybe this get-together was just drinks after a council meeting? But no, he'd said they were regulars, once a week for a couple of months. What was the connection? "And the fourth?" she asked.

"The little guy? That's Rishi Parmar. Surely you've seen his smiling face on the side of that monster truck he drives?" Jane laughed, nodding, and realizing she'd expected someone with such a big face and such a big truck to be a much bigger person. "Landscaping," her dad continued. "Every wealthy homeowner on both sides of the ridge. He's a wealthy man now himself." Joe lifted the heavy casserole dish into the wall oven, closed the door, and set the timer. "From what I can tell," he said, answering Jane's unspoken question, "it's some sort of little investment club. Nothing to do with City Council at all. And lucky for me, Cedars is the haunt they've chosen for their weekly meetings."

Draining the last of her latté, Jane rose and forced herself into the hallway to take another look at the members of Rand Harbinsale's investment club. Madge Moody was handing identical sheaves of paper to each of the others, some sort of financial report, Jane supposed. She was particularly friendly with Rishi Parmar, leaning against him and laughing at something he said. Looking pleased, he took the encouragement, mustered another witticism, and had her clapping her hands with glee. Gordon "Buzz" Gunnarson was drinking, all right, and seeming to offer toasts all around, but by the looks of the empty glasses on the table, he was managing only one for every two of Rand's.

The front door opened again in a rush of sound, Rand's head popped up, and Jane ducked back to avoid being seen. *What am I doing?* she wondered. *I have no reason to hide. Is it just that I want to avoid a conversation with Rand Harbinsale? He always seemed more keen to avoid* me *than the other way around* ... A sudden thought occurred to her. "Dad, does Mr. Harbinsale know you're my dad?" she asked. "I mean, would he connect me to the restaurant?" *He wouldn't come here if he knew,* she was thinking. *Not in a million years.*

"I don't suppose so, Jane," Joe confirmed as he measured out honey for more *baklava*. "I've certainly never said anything to him about you." He paused for a moment, thinking. "I gave him my business card once, but of course I go by 'Youssof Rahi' here." He smiled. "Authenticity, you know."

"Good," Jane nodded. "Would it be okay if we kept it that way?" She knew her dad would think her request had to do with Jake. But something else was tickling the back of her brain, and until she figured out what it was, she preferred to keep the advantage of anonymity.

Stepping back into the hallway, she peered around the corner and discovered that the latest arrival had seated himself with the city councilors. It was Cedar's Ridge Police Chief Brian Emery. Effie brought the Chief a coffee and a slice of *baklava*—"Compliments of the house, sir!"—and he took a moment to ask after Elias and their children before turning back to the conversation at the table.

Jane sighed, thinking it was probably time to stop acting like a spy without a mission and get home to the kitties. Just then, Chief Emery stood and motioned for Rand Harbinsale to follow. In a dim enclave at the back of the restaurant, out of earshot of the others, the Chief rested his hand on Rand's shoulder and spoke to him in low, earnest tones. Rand stood the intimacy as long as he could and then, casually extricating himself from the Chief's hand, let out a sharp laugh and said loudly, "Damn kids! They'll turn up. Good of you, Chief, but I wouldn't waste too much more police time on this. Elias! A glass of your best Scotch, neat, for the good man in blue, here!"

"No, thanks, Rand," Chief Emery answered. Rand's back was to her, but Jane could see both sympathy and confusion playing across the police chief's face. "I'm still on duty. And you take it easy there yourself!" He grinned and made as if to clap Rand on the back, then appeared to change his mind. "You got a ride home tonight?"

"What? Oh, absolutely. Eh, Buzz?" Rand nodded at Gordon Gunnarson, who looked from Rand to the Chief and nodded back.

"Well, all right then, I'll be on my way." Chief Emery retrieved his hat from the booth and headed for the door. "Goodnight, all. Goodnight, Effie, Elias. Thanks again." And he was gone.

"Jane, in or out, please. You're in the way there." Her mom brushed past her, carrying a stack of serviettes and stir sticks to the bar. Jane retreated to the kitchen, snatched up her bag and turned to give her dad a hug goodbye. It was way past time to go. Her mom appeared again in the doorway. "Plans for the weekend?"

"Yeah, Cultus, remember?" Jane replied. "We're leaving right after school tomorrow. I thought . . ." She paused. "You guys were going to try to come for one of the days, right?"

"Oh, Jane, I'm sorry," her dad replied, busy at the grill. "We got a huge booking for the holiday Monday and we'll be all weekend getting ready."

"Later in the season, maybe, Jane," her mom added. "Summer. We'll take a real little holiday. Hey, Joe?"

He turned and smiled, nodding, his hands folding the triangular *sfiha* pies automatically. "It's been a long time, hasn't it, Janey? The Ray family could use a holiday."

Brilliant deduction, dad, she thought. *More like, the Ray family could use some therapy.* "Okay, well, see you later then. Or, I guess, next week some time."

"Wear your sunscreen, Jane!"

"Do you need any money?"

"Yes, mom. No thanks, dad. Bye."

Seconds later, Jane slammed the car door and started

up the engine, revving it a few times just for the sake of making some noise. She still had homework to do before she could go to bed. Oh, and she had to pack for Cultus. Minnie would be a big help with that. She grinned, imagining the little tabby selecting toiletries and folding clothes. Home. Well, at least the lights would be on this time.

She swung the car backwards into the dark alley, shifted into first gear and was about to hit the gas when another car made a wide reverse sweep from the other side of the lot, its headlights swinging around to catch her full in the face, blinding her. She slammed on the breaks and sat immobilized, desperately hoping the other driver could see better than she could. There was a screech of tires as the other driver gunned his engine and roared past her in a cloud of smoke, missing her by inches. A blue-black BMW. She knew that car. And she'd recognized the man at the wheel, too. It was Rand Harbinsale.

8

EARLY MORNING VISITOR

JANE WOKE BEFORE THE OTHERS and lay in her bunk, knees up, eyes closed, hands folded behind her head, listening. It was the sound of Cultus Lake. The sound of her childhood. The underscore of sixteen summers, a raw melody lit with top notes of tastes and sights and smells and textures: the sweet tang of that stick of bubblegum that came with each pack of collector cards; the exact weight of wet sand in Amy's red plastic sandcastle bucket; the crackle of the blue and white paper wrappers that held Mike's balsawood gliders; the rumble and thunk of a can of cream soda falling like a pinball through the pop machine in the laundry hut; the waspy whine of go-karts on the track at the midway; the early-morning light pressing through goldenrod drapes in the cabin her family used to own, signaling that a new day had begun, that anything was possible.

It was the sound of crows.

They'd been up since 4:30 that Saturday morning, and Jane with them. It was earlier in the season—and there were more of them—than she remembered from previous years. The young were calling for food, the elders were calling to tell each other of good foraging and easy scavenging, calling to warn of enemies sighted in treetops, calling just to call. Depending on what you thought of crows, the calls might sound harsh, raucous, even violent. To Jane, crows were harbingers of summer, and their calls sounded like freedom.

There was a rustling in the bunk across from her, and Jane opened one eye to watch Amy roll onto her side, shucking off blanket and sheet in the process. She came perilously close to the edge of the bunk, and Jane snapped awake, ready to reach across and save her sleeping friend from falling to the floor. But just in time, Amy sank back against the far wall with a small snuffle, and Jane relaxed, stifling a giggle. It was already warm—the day would be hot—and the air in the small room was heavy and close. She could hear Flory breathing steadily in the bunk below her. The orderly girl wouldn't have moved a muscle since falling asleep the night before. The caahing outside intensified, and Jane turned to look through the small window as a duel broke out in midair between two crows laying claim to the same silver gum wrapper. Jane wondered how anyone could sleep through such noise.

"Somebody make it *stop*!" Amy's arms were folded across her face in a futile attempt to block out light and sound. Jane grabbed the pillow from beneath her head and tossed it across the small divide at her groggy friend. "Oof!" Amy curled into a ball, caterpillar-like, and moaned. "The sky is falling!"

Jane glanced down at the alarm clock. It was only just past 5:00 a.m. "Time for our run, Chicken Little!" she teased in a whisper, trying not to wake Flory. "Rise and shine!"

Amy curled tighter. "I dreamed I ran. Doesn't that count?"

There was a sharp rap at the window, just inches from her face, and Jane whirled, startled. Nothing. But there had been something. What? A branch, maybe? Those of the closest tree, a beech, formed a leafy green round, like a child's drawing of a tree. Nothing there to brush her window. But something had.

"Amy . . . *Ame*!" Jane spoke in an insistent whisper now. "Wake up. Did you see something at the window just now?"

"I saw nothing," Amy muttered, hugging her arms tighter around her head. "Not my fault. Nothing to do with it."

"Amy, I'm serious," Jane pressed, extending a leg across the space between the beds with a mind to kicking her friend into action if necessary. She almost fell off her bunk when the sharp tap came again, followed by a frantic scrabbling sound. Yanking her leg in and up, she curled into the fetal position, rolled left, and came face to beak with a large black crow. Her eyes went wide, and the crow, struggling to maintain its hold on the narrow sill, cocked its head, stared back at her, and blinked.

"Yaghh!" she blurted, then clapped a hand to her mouth. The sound, and her sudden motion, scared the crow from its precarious perch, and it lofted itself into the air and flew out of sight.

"Did you *see* that?" she intoned in hushed awe. In all her sixteen summers of listening to crows at Cultus Lake, she had never been visited by one. She looked over; Amy was awake now, eyes and mouth wide open in surprise.

"That I saw," she answered, nodding slowly. "Had I not seen, I would not have believed." They were still whispering. Somehow, Flory still slept.

Despite the warmth of the room, Jane shivered and drew her blanket back up to her chin. The rattling caahs were loud and urgent and constant now, and Jane ducked instinctively as one noisy gathering flew down from the trees and over the cabin, lending their voices to the cacophony. She heard small taps overhead, like impatient fingernails on a tabletop. Part of the gathering had taken to the roof of the cabin and was leading the call from there.

There were more crows now, Jane was sure, than there had been five or ten years ago. More here. More in the city. Through the winter and spring in Cedar's Ridge she had watched as hundreds upon thousands of crows took to the skies each day at dusk, traveling from every corner of the city to congregate at the junction of Tellington Road and the highway. The sky was a mass of moving shadows, black on blue, and the small silhouettes filled the tops of the skeletal trees like dark ornaments, living, breathing, watching. Five to eight thousand, the bird watchers estimated. The largest gathering in the province. Right there in Cedar's Ridge.

The obvious explanation was their ability to adapt. As the city sprawled and the wilds diminished, vulnerable species disappeared, and the animals that fared best in the company of humans proliferated. They borrowed human homes for lookouts and their litter for nests, and ate their garbage for food. They thrived. And noisily. Crows didn't sneak around, apologizing for their burgeoning presence. They took the trees, skies, roads, and private yards as they wished, and all the while, they got closer.

Close enough to tap on my window. Jane couldn't help but think that with their growing numbers and their noisy calls, they were trying to say something, get a message through to human beings. As though they knew people were too dense to get the message through pretty feathers and sweet song. It was human nature: things have to get ugly before we'll listen.

Jane felt rather than heard the gathering lift from the lakeside trees on the far side of the cabin. It was as if the sky moved. The calling had abated, but now it crescendoed again, urgent, discordant, and every crow in every tree seemed to call an answer as the gathering approached. The tearing caahs were a wall of sound.

Suddenly it stopped and the world went silent. Jane heard Flory rise upright in bed with a gasp. With a great rush of air like the sweep of an owl's wing, every crow in every tree rose up to join the approaching group and passed directly over the cabin above Jane's window. Hundreds of black shapes, a hundred thousand feathers blocking the sun. For just a moment, the sunny room went dark.

"What is it?" Flory cried from the bunk below Jane. Amy had thrown herself across the small space between bunk beds and she and Jane knelt side by side at the window, hands braced on the wall, staring at the sky. Blue sky framed by cedars and pine, the lake behind reflecting bright morning sun on a warm, fresh Saturday in May.

"What is it?" Flory said again, this time from the ladder, where she stood peering up over the top bunk and trying to see out the window. "What's wrong?"

The three friends exchanged glances. Wordlessly, all three looked back to the window and beyond it to the perfect new day.

"I don't know," answered Jane.

I don't know.

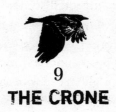

9

THE CRONE

JANE, AMY, AND FLORY WERE in Logan's Market gathering groceries for that night's meal, and Jane was telling her two best friends about her encounter with Rand Harbinsale and his fellow councilors at Cedars the night before. "My dad thinks it's some kind of investment club."

"Reminds me of one of those bad religious jokes," Amy quipped, reaching across Jane and plucking two bundles of asparagus from the neat mounds of produce. "You know, so a golfer, a barber, a gardener, and a landscaper walk into a bar . . ." She snorted. "Or maybe that *Sesame Street* song—'One of These Things is Not Like the Other.'" The spray misters came on. She plopped a dripping bunch of baby carrots into her basket and moved on to the next aisle.

"It does make you wonder what they all have in common," Jane agreed as she hefted melons and nectarines, testing their ripe-and-juicy quotient.

"Drugs," Amy tossed off from behind a pyramid of tinned tomatoes. Jane could see her in one of Logan's new security mirrors, red curls flying as she glanced both ways before sneaking a malt ball from the bulk bin. "I hear there's decent money in it."

"Give me a break," Jane said, laughing in spite of herself. She added bananas, kiwis, and strawberries to her basket. "If you'd seen this fussy little Moody woman, you'd guess they had shares in china figurines or were trading in quilting fabrics or something, not drugs."

"It's always the quiet ones," Amy sang in lilting tones, dancing now in time to *Caribbean Queen* as it crackled through the store's ancient speakers. Jane reminded herself to bring Mr. Logan a CD next time she came in. Something a little more up to date. Even the nineties would be nice.

"I'm going to be seeing a lot of Rand Harbinsale and the city councilors this summer," Flory interjected almost shyly. "Maybe I can find out what they're up to."

After a short silence, Jane whooped, understanding. "You got it! Flory! You got the job!" Flory's eyes shone like two black stones as she nodded, yes. She had applied for a position as a summer research intern with Cedar's Ridge City Hall, along with a few hundred other students, many of them older and more experienced than she was. It had been a long shot, but in the end, the girl's professional demeanor and her awareness of the issues the city was tackling had won over the interview panel.

"I'm going to be working with two departments:

city parks and environmental operations," Flory explained. "Councilor Harbinsale's office is just down the hall from my desk. It will be fun to have a little extra 'research' to do!" She grinned, keen for the covert challenge, then lowered her voice to a whisper. "My guess is it's a gardening club, and they're purchasing rare plant species from around the world. Any other theories? We could place bets!"

"I still say it's drugs," Amy muttered, miffed that her theory had been rejected out of hand. She reached over the shelf of canned legumes to hand Jane a bag of dark chocolate chunks for the fondue. "Hey, tell me, why am I the only one who has to lock lips with Ellson Farquharson just to make a few bucks this summer?"

"What?" Jane cried.

"Ewww!" Flory squealed.

"Exactly," Amy shot back from the far aisle. "Apparently summer interns at the provincial lab have to have their first aid ticket. I mean, what do they think is going to happen in a *lab*, for crying out loud? It doesn't get any safer than science!" Jane and Flory exchanged a glance, thinking back to exploding green foam and an indescribable smell.

"Mr. Voted-Most-Likely-to-be-Polygamous got hired as a lifeguard at the outdoor pool—big surprise, like, maybe the all-year tan helped?—and has to take a refresher first aid course," Amy continued. "*My* course," she wailed. "He's already talking about how we can be partners for CPR and mouth-to-mouth." She shuddered. "I'm worried he's going to come out with some of this stuff when Ben's around!"

"Ben would beat him up, I think," Flory said in a hushed voice, her eyes wide. Jane nodded her agreement. The scene would not be pretty. *Ellson* would need first aid if Ben caught wind of what he'd been saying.

Amy came tearing into the produce aisle and caught Flory up in a bear hug. "Flory, you're a genius!" she shouted. "I'll make sure Ben accidentally overhears Ellson's plans as soon as we're back at school." She strode away, grooving happily to Thomas Dolby's *She Blinded Me With Science*, circa 1982.

"Jane, your job with the UWRC starts soon, doesn't it?" Flory asked, relieved to change the subject and sorry to have been such an inspiration to Amy.

Jane nodded, lowering her basket to the floor to give her arm a break. "End of June. Evie said yesterday the sponsor had already contacted her about my super-hero-mobile. So I guess I'll be out on the road rescuing animals and spreading the word about wildlife protection in just a few weeks!" She did a little dance, unable to contain her excitement. She could still hardly believe the opportunity that had come her way after less than a year as a volunteer with the little wildlife hospital.

"More important topic . . ." Amy was back, full basket suspended from one arm and a watermelon perched on the opposite shoulder. "What are you two wearing to the dance tonight? First one of the season! Gotta send the right message to all the new summer boys!"

Jane put her hands on her hips and tried to look disapproving. "Uh-huh, and what message would that be, O committed girlfriend of honor-defending Ben Tremblay?" she inquired archly.

"Oh, you know," Amy teased. "Welcome to Cultus Lake . . . c'mon in, the water's warm!"

Jane shook her head, laughing. Summer boys. Why couldn't she be content with a summer boy? What more was it that she wanted? She was only seventeen. This was the time for summer boys, short and sweet romances, temporary flings. Nothing serious. Just for fun. But she'd discovered with Jake Harbinsale that her feelings ran deeper than that, and that as much as it hurt when things hadn't worked out, it was *that* kind of connection she wanted. Nothing less really interested her.

Amy was describing the iridescent blue platform sandals she'd discovered at Shopping City, and Flory told them how she'd found the exact pink babydoll dress she'd fallen in love with in a magazine. Jane realized that between her unsettling night at Cedars and her rushed packing job this morning, she'd forgotten to bring her skirt. Jeans, a tank top, and her flip-flops were somehow going to have to send the "right message" to the new summer boys. She grinned at the thought, deciding she didn't care in the least.

As they gathered up the rest of the items on Mrs. MacGillivray's shopping list, they spoke again of the odd events of the early morning. "It was like a dream," Jane said of the startling visitation and the passing of the crows, "you know, that same weird real-but-not-real feeling, except we all saw the same thing. We were all awake."

"There is more than one way to dream."

The voice seemed to come from inside Jane's head, and it was a moment before she realized someone had actually spoken. She glanced up at the security mirror in time to see a figure gliding away from the far side of the produce tables and retreating down the dry goods aisle. Shorter than she remembered. Silver streaks now in the mane of coppered black. Jeans and a plaid work shirt replaced the flowing, fringed robes. But unmistakable nonetheless. It was the Crone.

"That'll be fifteen dollars, seventy-seven, if you please, ma'am!" Arnie Logan punched myopically at the keys protruding from the round belly of the old cash register, and slowly loaded groceries into paper bags. "Now, perhaps the girls will be kind enough to help you out with these. You certainly are going through the canned soup and cold cuts these days, Audrey!" *Audrey,* Jane thought. *So she had a name.* "Some newfangled diet I haven't heard about?" Mr. Logan chuckled heartily, patting change into his customer's outstretched hand.

Jane stood nervously behind the Crone, basket in hand, wondering whether she should say something before the woman left the store. Had she been mistaken? She'd been sure the voice was real. Between dreams and dead crows, feathered visitors and mysterious voices, though, the last couple of days had been enough to make her doubt her own senses. But something had compelled her to follow the Crone all the way through Logan's to the checkout counter. And that same something had compelled Amy and Flory to fall into line behind her. She glanced back, catching sight of Amy's raised eyebrows and Flory's nervous frown. In all the years they'd been coming to Cultus, in all the years they'd known the Crone, never once had they spoken to her. Nor, for that matter, had she ever spoken to them. Jane cleared her throat.

"You got my message." It was a statement rather than a question and came before Jane had had a chance to speak. Again, the voice seemed to arise from inside her head. Jane stared wide-eyed at the Crone's back, then whirled around, looking beseechingly to Amy and Flory for some clue as to what was going on. Both shrugged helplessly, their eyes as wide as hers.

When she turned back, the Crone had turned, too, and stood facing her. Mouth upturned in a small smile. Broad, high cheekbones. Lines that sketched out a lifetime of laughter and grief. And eyes Jane remembered from years and years ago—childlike, ancient, ageless. They twinkled up at her now, mischief and a question in them. She spoke again, and this time Jane saw with relief that her lips moved quite normally as she did so.

"You *are* the Ray girl? The one who was on TV last year? Fighting that oil company and saving the animals? 'S'at you?"

Jane nodded, unable to find her voice.

"Thought so!" the Crone said, folding her hands and smiling as though everything had been cleared up. "That's why I sent Crow this morning. I decided it was time to invite you over for a visit." She lifted her bags from the counter and started toward the door. "Settle up with Arnie. I'll wait outside."

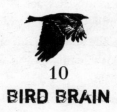

10
BIRD BRAIN

They walked along the shoreline path to the trailer park at the northeast end of the lake—neat rows of mobile homes and miniature gardens surrounded by woods, backed by train tracks, and ambitiously named the Mountainview Country Club. The Crone led the way, empty-handed, whistling, and Jane, Amy, and Flory followed carrying her groceries as well as their own. About half way between Logan's and the trailer park, a large crow swooped down from a copse of tall trees, its ragged "caah-caahs" sounding like a battle cry as it made straight for the little party. Terrified of birds, Flory screamed, dropped her bags, and stood immobilized in the path. Drawing level with Jane, the crow circled above her, a hundred, then fifty, then twenty feet in the air. Unsure as to whether she was just imagining things or genuinely under attack, Jane ran up the path ahead of the Crone. Turning, she jogged backwards, shading her eyes with her hand as she scanned the sky for her would-be assailant. She sensed the Crone giving her a hard stare. Then the older woman turned as well, lifted her left hand into the air, and changed her whistling tune.

Coasting on a slight eddy that blew across the lake from the southwest, the crow was a black cutout shape on cloudless blue sky—broad wingspan at near-perfect right angles to its body and tipped with feathers that looked remarkably like fingers, its short fan of a tail trimmed almost square across. The crow flapped twice, three times, propelling itself forward and down. At the last second, it angled its body tail-downward, wings thrust forward to slow its flight, and then it extended its legs, toes flexed, like landing gear, alighting without any further negotiations on the Crone's outstretched hand.

"This is Crow," the Crone said. "She's a friend of mine." Jane and Amy crowded around the strange pair, and even Flory, hanging back at a safe distance, was drawn in by curiosity. The woman stroked the feathers on the bird's crown and breast, and the animal emitted a series of gurgles and chortles that expressed in very clear terms her affection for her human friend and her delight in being petted. "Known her about seventeen years, and she was full grown back then, so she could be even older than that. Older than you girls, I'll bet!"

That phrase, *She's a friend of mine*, called a memory to the surface that Jane hadn't thought of for years. The sprawling cherry tree near the entrance to the trailer park, in its branches a square wooden platform used by probably hundreds of children over the years as their secret hiding place. She, Amy, and Flory used to climb into the tree and spend whole afternoons on that platform, playing games they'd invented, reading mystery books, lying on their backs staring up at the sky through gnarled branches, feasting on warm, ripe cherries. Once in a while, Jane's mom would let them take her field glasses into the tree, and they would spy on the occupants of the trailer park, filling notebooks with their detailed observations. Most often, Jane watched the Crone.

Had it been Amy's dad who first called her that? The little girls had heard "crow," not knowing the other word, and had called her "the crow" until Mr. MacGillivray had laughingly corrected them. Jane made a mental note now to tell him they'd learned her real name.

She'd stood out, that was for sure, at the lakeside, in the village, at the Community Hall, in her dark, floor-length robes, her rings and necklaces set with large polished stones, the sheath of black hair that hung to her waist. Jane had greatly admired that hair, and the veined turquoises and bottomless ambers she wore, the brilliantly dyed clothes she hung on her line, so different from the beiges and whites flapping behind the other trailers, and the way she whistled and sang whenever she walked through the village. There had been children who made fun of her, Jane remembered, pointing and laughing, calling her crazy, not bothering even to do it behind her back. Really, though, had Jane's secret spying been any better? She'd felt sorry for the Crone as a child, for the fact that she lived in a trailer when her own family and friends had nice cabins. She'd felt sorry for all the trailer park people for that reason. Four years ago, her family had had to sell their cabin because of financial troubles; even a trailer would be unaffordable now. She suddenly wondered whether any of the trailer park people felt sorry for *her*.

The afternoon Jane was thinking of, they'd been watching the Crone pick wildflowers along the path just outside the trailer park. Jane had been eight that year, or maybe nine. She could recall wondering why the woman chose all yellow and gold blossoms and their leaves, and not the delicate pink ones as she would have done. The field glasses were powerful enough to let her see a bee floating above the center of one of the blooms in the Crone's hand, its legs dipping down to gather what nectar it could before the Crone began to move toward a thicket of blackberry bushes at the edge of the woods.

Suddenly, the Crone had dropped to a crouch, her head moving forward and disappearing from view. The rest of her followed. It was as if the drape of the blackberry canes formed a kind of cave, and the Crone was hiding inside. That, at least, was the conclusion the girls had come to. Rapidly, they passed the field glasses back and forth, but none of them could see through the thick tangle of blackberries. After ten minutes, they'd been about to give up and turn the glasses on Mr. Lollyamble and his pet pig, when out of the blackberry thicket rose a shiny black crow, the stem of a single yellow flower in its bill. The girls had waited, breath held, for the Crone to reemerge as well, but she never did. The afternoon shadows grew long, and soon they could hear their mothers calling them back to the cabins for dinner.

As Jane stared now at Crone and Crow together, she wondered if she was looking at the solution to that mystery. Or perhaps yet another mystery.

Crow left the Crone's hand and took to the air again to accompany them home. Jane saw her light on the branch of a maple tree and rob another bird's nest of a twig. Taking off again, Crow dropped the twig in midair, its fall broken only slightly by the breeze, and then swooped like a fighter pilot to catch it before it hit the ground. "Holy crow!" Amy hollered. "She's playing!" Sure enough, Crow repeated the trick twice more before tiring of the game and looking for a new one. "Did you teach her to do that?"

"She's *my* teacher," the Crone answered with a broad smile. "I can't teach that birdbrain nothin'! Anyway, she's already smarter than most people I know." As if to demonstrate, Crow flew to the top of the tool shed next to one of the cabins lining the trail, its aluminum roof gleaming in the late-afternoon sun. Launching herself head first off the peak, she slid down its slope on her back, a raucous black toboggan, coming to a stop in the upturn of the roof's ledge. The girls burst out laughing. "She'll be sorry," the Crone said, laughing too. "Bet that roof's hot."

By some miracle of avian acrobatics, Crow simultaneously flipped herself upright and launched herself once more into the air, this time aiming for a discarded popsicle stick she'd spotted on the path ahead of them. Grasping one end of the stick in her beak, she hopped over to the softer earth at the edge of the path and began to dig. Once she'd struck gold, she dropped the stick and plucked the unfortunate beetle up in her bill.

"H-hey!" Amy spluttered. "That's impossible!" She bent forward, staring at the intrepid Crow, who was staring back. "You can't use tools . . . only primates use tools!"

Flory shook her head. "Keep up, Ame. Corvids, too. 'Birdbrain' isn't an insult any more, it's a compliment!" The Crone cackled her assent.

They had reached the gates of Mountainview Country Club, the 1960s-style turquoise-and-white sign looking jaunty with a fresh coat of paint, and the Crone ushered them through, waving familiarly to the security guard as they passed. Pointing to an old pine behind the first row of trailers—one of the few tall trees left on park property—she said, "Her nest's up there. That's her tree. No eggs this year, though. First time. She's a widow now, just like me." She turned down that first row and stopped at the third trailer, white with blue trim much like all the others, neat rows of flowers lining the front yard and a barrel by the stairs brimming with a lush water garden. And then she opened the door and ushered them in.

Inside, the Crone's trailer was nothing like any of the others. Nothing like anything Jane had ever seen. She took in the narrow, knotted birch sapling panels that covered the walls, their light color making the whole room brighter and larger-seeming than it was. One long wall was paneled normally, straight up and down, but on the opposite length, the saplings had been bent into a gentle curve at their height, so that they arched across the top of the room, their ends meeting the join of wall and ceiling on the far side. Jane caught her breath in recognition: the whole room was shaped like the wing of a bird.

The furnishings were made of wood, hand-carved shapes designed to fit both the room and the human body, and the walls were hung with carvings of bears and birds, weavings of various sizes and shapes, and intricate spiders'-web designs set in silver hoops, large versions of the earrings Jane had seen the Crone wear. Everything was spare, and beautiful because it belonged. There was nothing extra, nothing missing. Even to Jane, who had never been in such a place, it felt like home.

A moment later, Crow landed on the ledge of the open window, called a quick greeting, and flew to her perch. The Crone took Jane's hand and sifted something into it. "For Crow," she said gruffly, indicating to Jane to hold her hand out to the bird. Crow's bill tickled Jane's palm as she selected sunflower seeds and kernels of corn from the mound of treats the girl held out. She shucked the seed hulls easily with her strong jaw and dropped them to the tray below her perch, making small rooking noises as she savored the meat inside. Jane had to keep reminding herself that this was a wild animal and not a pet. The perch, the tray, the fact that the bird was contentedly eating out of her hand—the fact that they were *inside* the Crone's trailer—all seemed to say "tame." But she'd seen proof the bird was wild.

Amy and Flory had been gawking their way around the room, openmouthed and unembarrassed. For years, the three of them had imagined what the home of "the crazy Crone" might look like. Every guess had been wrong. With Crow's arrival, Flory screamed again and ran to crouch behind the kitchen counter. Amy turned, hands on hips, and affected a pout. "Why does that bird like Jane so much? Don't we get to feed her, too?" She made as if to reach for the perch.

The Crone stilled her with a serious look. "Crow'll take food from you, I'm sure," she answered Amy. She emitted a small chuckle. "She'd take food from anyone." Her face grew stern again. "You just might not want to take what she has to give *you*."

Jane froze. Slowly, she pulled her hand away from Crow's searching bill, eliciting a series of annoyed squawks from the frustrated bird. "What she has to give . . . What are you talking about?" Her voice sounded rude to her own ears, but she didn't care. "Is she giving something to *me?*" Jane felt her heart thump in her chest, and the hand holding the mound of seeds and nuts was trembling. Maybe everybody had been right years ago. Maybe the woman *was* crazy. Or evil.

A whistling sound started and rose to a high-pitched shriek. Rather than answering Jane, the Crone moved to the kitchen, stepping gently around Flory as she turned the burner off under the kettle and slowly filled the teapot. Something about her unhurried, deliberate movements calmed Jane. But only a little.

The Crone placed the teapot and four pottery mugs on a round wooden tray and carried them into the big room, where she set them down on a low table and then sat herself down as well. "You already have it, Jane," she finally replied, holding the teapot by its handle and spout and swirling the contents. "She's only been followin' you around to tell you you'd better be ready to use it." For a moment, the only sound in the room was the familiar burble of tea as it filled the mugs.

Flory stood up then, and the three girls found their voices at the same time. "Have what?" they said in unison. "Use *what?*"

The Crone looked up from pouring tea and blinked, as if surprised they didn't know. Then she set the tea things back down on the tray and put her hands on her knees, looking to Flory, then Amy, and finally to Jane. At last, she smiled her broad smile, and Jane felt that same sense of calm again, resting side by side with her fear of what the woman would say. She felt like a game show contestant who'd just won some mystery prize that was going to change her life forever. Only she was pretty sure she was going to wish she'd picked door number two. "I already have what?" she repeated, almost in a whisper.

"Crow medicine."

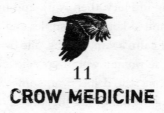

11
CROW MEDICINE

"LISTEN, MRS. CRO . . . uh, Audrey. Mrs. Audrey," Amy's hands were on her hips and her eyes flashed dangerously. "It's been really great hauling your groceries home for you and meeting your pet bird and everything, but I think we really oughta be going now. Isn't that right, Jane?" She yanked her head toward the door.

"Thank you very much for your hospitality," Flory put in graciously, with a nod toward the full mugs of tea still steaming on the polished tree stump that served as a coffee table. She kept her eyes on Crow as she inched discreetly toward the door.

Jane wasn't sure what made her do it, but the impulse was strong and clear. She reached forward, lifted a mug of tea from the table and took a sip. Peppermint. To clear the mind, settle the nerves. Looking directly at her friends, she said, "I think I'll stay, actually. Go ahead. I'll be back in time to help with dinner."

Amy's eyebrows shot up to her hairline, and Flory emitted a small "Oh!"

"Yeah, so, see you in an hour or so!" Jane said, trying to sound more confident than she felt.

There was silence, and then, "An hour," Amy said with finality, pointing a finger at Jane. She turned again to face the Crone: "An hour," she repeated. She hefted their groceries. "Let's go, Flory." Flory turned and opened the door, letting in the slanted rays of late-afternoon sun and letting herself out. Amy glanced again at Jane before stepping outside and closing the door behind her.

The trailer went still and silent. Dust motes swirled in the air, made visible by the streaks of sunlight glancing in through the front window. Jane took another sip of her tea. *I'm the crazy one here*, she thought, hoping she looked engrossed in her sipping and not as though she were already plotting an escape. *I should've left while I had the chance.*

"You can still go if you want," the Crone said, sipping her own tea and not looking up. Jane almost choked. "I only thought it might help if you understood." The room was silent again, and Jane felt that now-familiar sense of calm steal through her as she took in the Crone's words. It was, she realized, the same feeling she had when she was trying to help a wild bird that was struggling with fear as she held it in her hands. She'd always wondered whether she managed to transmit any of her own calm to the bird. Now she knew. This peace she felt was coming from the woman across from her, and right now, she was the frightened bird. She made her decision and sat down to face the Crone.

"By the way, please call me Audrey." Audrey smiled, meeting her eyes.

Ah. So she'd known that, too. Jane blushed deeply, and then seeing the twinkle in those eyes, suddenly felt a laugh bubbling up from somewhere deep inside. She let it out, and Audrey answered it with a belly laugh of her own. The two put down their tea mugs and laughed til their sides ached.

Wiping her eyes, Audrey said, "You have good friends, Jane. They'd do anything for you. And vice-a-versa, I think, too. You chose well."

"Caah!" Crow called out her agreement, and flew from her perch to land on the back of Jane's chair.

"Crow chose well, too, yes," Audrey nodded at the bird, then looked at Jane. "You used her medicine just now, when your friends left and you decided to stay. Most people go their whole lives and never learn to make up their own minds, you know that? Little stuff, important stuff, they just do what somebody else wants 'em to do. Or whatever everybody else does. You're learnin' early. That's crow medicine. Or part of it, anyway." She took a long draught of her tea.

"And last year, when I saw you on TV, you were usin' it then, too." Jane glanced at her, suddenly remembering her words back at Logan's. She knew about the oil spill, then, and about Jane's role in bringing the culprit to justice. "Aren't too many who'll take a stand 'cause of some ducks." She grinned. "Or make fools of themselves in public for—well, for anything, never mind animals. That's when I knew you had it. Croooow medicine!" She drew the words out slow, like a song.

"What does that mean, medicine?" Jane frowned. "I thought medicine was just gross-tasting stuff you took when you got sick. But when you say it, it sounds like something else. Like something . . . good."

"Medicine is power," Audrey replied simply. "Your medicine tells you which way you're supposed to walk in life. Thing is, we don't walk our path alone. You have your friends, for instance," she said, nodding toward the door, "'Amy medicine' and 'Flory medicine' to protect you." She chuckled again. "You have your family. And animals, too." Jane nodded and smiled, thinking of Sweet Pea and Minnie curled like fiddleheads on either side of her in bed.

"And not just the ones you call pets," Audrey said, divining her thoughts. "Every animal carries its own power, its own medicine," she explained, tracing the rings in the polished tree-stump table with a small, worn hand, "and if an animal is your guide, then you have that animal's medicine to help you on your path."

"And I have crow medicine?" Jane asked tentatively.

"Crow, yes. And probably others, too," Audrey answered. "If there's animals you keep meetin' up with over and over again in your life, chances are, they're your medicine animals. Pay attention to those ones." She smiled, tilted her head back, and drained the last of her tea, then looked directly at Jane. "But today, we talk about Crow, because I know Crow the best." She smiled, almost wistfully. "I have crow medicine, too. So I can tell you somethin' about yourself."

Later, when Jane was telling Amy and Flory what transpired in Audrey's trailer that afternoon, she would say that the older woman's voice had changed then, had seemed to come from somewhere deeper than larynx and lungs, and that her appearance, too, had altered as she spoke, becoming by turns youthful and aged, innocent and wise.

Crow flies the course between the spirit world and the earth walk, carrying messages from the living to the dead, and from the dead to the living. She wears the black robes of the law—not worldly law but spiritual law—and it is her task to uphold the proper order of things as it was set forth in the beginning. When balance has been disrupted, Crow will be there, working to make things right. Her appearance foretells great change, and you will need to see with different eyes and know with a different mind if you are to understand what is required of you.

Some say she made this world, and everything in it, and knows every person she made, and each petal on every flower. Some say she stole the light from the heaven-dwellers and gave it to the earth-walkers so that they would know the beauty she had made for them. Some say she brought them water so they would not thirst, and sent the salmon so they would not hunger. For it is understood that when you have brought something into being, you are responsible for it for all its days.

Crow has friends in the raven, and in the squirrel and the wolf, but her path is difficult and so there are many turns of the earth and cycles of the moon during which she flies alone. She has not the sing-song voice of other birds, and she tells not the sweet tales they tell. Her voice is harsh, and her stories are often so, as well. They are always true, yes, but the truth does not win her friends or gather companions to her on her path. At times, she calls til her voice is hoarse searching for someone who will listen to what she has to say.

Those who walk with Crow on their shoulder may be rebels, tricksters, jokers, and shapeshifters, outspoken about those things others would prefer to ignore and willing to dress the fool if necessary to cut through the heavy haze of illusion and bring the truth to light. And they will do so, whatever the consequences. Their lives are not quite their own, as Crow calls on them often to leave the comfort of their individual lives behind and act for the good of the whole community. When they do meet a friend on the path, they are loyal for life.

Though she flies only with whom she chooses, Crow calls us all to defend and protect that which we cherish. Those who refuse her call will find themselves ever unable to distinguish between real and unreal, and will live as

though from behind a veil, separated from life by com-
fortable illusion. Those who need her medicine will find
her at crossroads, in the dark places, and at the gateway
between living and dying. Those who seek her will always
find her, and she will show them the way home. She has
brought us all into being and set us free and will watch
over us for all our days.

Audrey stopped speaking, and Crow took up where she left off, setting up a raucous clamor that brought Audrey to her feet. Jane blinked, hardly sure of where she was.

If Audrey's tale had been meant to "help her understand" the events of the past three days, it had not; it had merely raised more questions. Jane had told her nothing about her rescue of the fledgling crow, or of the crows that had been killed and left at the wildlife center. But the woman seemed to have an intuition about things, about *Jane*. Or perhaps she had heard of the advance of West Nile Virus on television and surmised that anyone associated with a wild animal hospital would be impacted by the news. Still, that would mean a lot of assumptions about a whole lot of variables. And really, Audrey had simply bumped into her at Logan's, invited her home, and explained to Jane her understanding of the essence of crows. Simple as that.

But for what? What possible use could Jane have for such myths and fairy tales, fascinating as they were, in a world governed by science, facts, disease, and *real* medicine? And yet why was some part of her absolutely sure she'd just heard something true?

Crow medicine. And she was supposed to have it. Same as Audrey. Same as the Crone. Croney old Jane Ray. She could hear Amy now; this was *not* going to improve her score with the guys at Cedar's Ridge High.

Supressing a smile, she looked up to find Audrey pulling a small, silver metal ring, a pencil, and a slip of paper from a drawer in the side table. The older woman wrote out a short message in shaky block letters, then rolled it up tightly and slipped it inside a tiny tube soldered onto the side of the ring. As if on cue, Crow lofted herself over Jane's head and landed on Audrey's outstretched hand, where she submitted to having the ring fastened around her left leg.

As she lifted Crow to the windowsill, Audrey said, "Take it to Eunice!" Crow tipped forward across the sill and was gone.

"Oh!" Jane cried. "Crow's a carrier pigeon! Er, carrier crow."

Audrey laughed. "All crows are messengers. Just that some take their job a little more seriously!"

Jane helped Audrey clear the teapot and mugs and then checked her watch: fifty-two minutes. Almost time to go, unless she wanted to see Amy burst through that door and take Audrey down in a football tackle. "You know, um, Audrey," she stammered, "I'm not sure I understood everything you said. I've never heard about animals having medicine before. Or about people having the powers of different animals. I'm trying to get it, I really am, but I feel kind of like I'm, well, missing something." She was afraid she sounded rude, or ungrateful, but she wanted something from this woman that would make everything fall into place. She felt as though the events of the past three days were random pieces of a puzzle, and she'd swallowed her fears and stayed to hear what Audrey had to say because she'd hoped her words might solve that puzzle. Instead, they'd turned out to be just more pieces, and Jane had no more idea now of how they all fit together than before she arrived. If there was something she'd missed, or something Audrey had forgotten to tell her, she wanted to find out now.

Audrey listened to Jane without interrupting, drying her dishes with care and putting them away. When Jane stopped speaking, she said casually, "School's good, right? Books, TV, hearin' stuff from your parents. Lots of ways to learn. But if you ask me, you never really get it til you live it. That's when you hope all that learnin' stuck, is when you're in the middle of things and you gotta use it." She paused, then looked up at Jane, her bright eyes serious, but kind. "You're gonna live it. Soon, I think. And when you're in the middle of it, this'll all make sense." She winked. "I hope."

The front door burst open and four small bodies hurled themselves at Audrey, yelling as though they meant to knock the walls down. Two boys and two girls, all dark-haired and bright-eyed, surrounded her like a cyclone, and she bent, laughing, to give each a bear hug and a quiet word before pushing them in the direction of the kitchen. They ran to the fridge, one yanked open the freezer door and each pulled out a pink-lemonade popsicle. Passing by her again like a parade, noise level still at rock-concert decibel levels, they bestowed four lemony kisses on her waiting cheek before barreling for the door. "Those two are my daughter's children," Audrey said to Jane, pointing, "and those two, my son's."

"Heyyyy Eunice!" Jane heard them yell as they clattered down the stairs, to be replaced by a cackling, bleach-haired woman in a citrus-fruit-print caftan and rollers, unlit cigarette held aloft to protect it from being knocked out of her hand.

"Glad to see you're keeping them in line, Audrey," Eunice said, cackling again. She narrowed her cackle to a thin stream of hoots as she lit her cigarette. "Disciplinarian you ain't!"

Audrey made a derisive noise in the back of her throat. "Discipline? Love and popsicles, I say. Who wants a grandma with more rules than school?" At that, Eunice narrowed her eyes as if trying to decide whether she'd just been insulted. After a moment, she shrugged and took a long drag on her cigarette.

"Don't smoke that thing in here, I always tell you!" Audrey said over her shoulder as she made her way to the back end of the trailer. "I gotta use the loo—all that tea. So, everybody on for poker tonight?" She disappeared into the bathroom and closed the door.

Eunice leaned toward Jane, lowering her voice conspiratorially and holding a hand up to her mouth. "Woman's got more money than God and she makes us play with pennies!" She lifted the cigarette to her mouth again, glanced toward the bathroom door, then went to the kitchen and ran it under the tap until it was soggy. "Won't go to the casino, won't go to bingo. Crotchety old cheapskate! I have no idea where she got it all, or what she plans to do with it. Mending rich people's fancy clothes for The Hudson's Bay Company, I don't think so! Me, I'd be outta here in a flash, buy me a fancy home in one of them neighborhoods, you know, with the cul-de-sacs. But not her. Oh, no! Says she saves it. I say, 'Who for? Your kids? They don't need it! They're just fine! It's yours,' I say. 'Enjoy it!' And you know what she says to me? Says, 'I'm savin' it for the Crow.' For that blasted bird! Can you believe that? I mean, what's *she* gonna do with it, build a nest?" Eunice laughed, and started to wheeze a little. "Can't you just see it? Great big nest made outta thousand-dollar bills? Now, that's when you know you're rich. Got enough money to build a nest outta thousand-dollar bills." Eunice "tsked" like she'd had a lot of practice making that sound. "You'd think she could up the stakes a little at poker."

Audrey emerged from the bathroom, glanced at

Eunice who was watching something out the window, and then winked at Jane. She'd heard every word. Surprised almost into a laugh, Jane found herself winking back. She glanced down at her watch again and was about to say goodbye when suddenly she remembered something. "Audrey, back at Logan's, you said something about dreaming, about there being more than one way to dream. What did you mean?"

Audrey nodded. "You gonna be at the fire tonight?"

"No," Jane said. "I'm going to the dance. Why?"

"Maybe you'll make it to the fire tonight," was all she answered.

Jane nodded at Eunice, who shrugged as she pulled another cigarette from her pack, then turned to Audrey, not sure what to say. "Well, um, thanks for . . . everything, I guess." *Wow, what an orator you are, Jane! Have you considered a career in politics?* She cringed inwardly at her own stunted social skills.

Audrey looked at her hard then, as if trying to gage exactly how much of "everything" had actually sunk in. Then her face softened and she smiled. "You are full." She bowed her head and closed her eyes for a moment. "I'm full, too."

Jane felt a lump rise in her throat, and tears stung the back of her eyes. Why did every word this woman uttered seem to say more than most people's whole conversations? "Well, goodbye, then," was all she managed in reply. She turned to go, but was surprised to see Audrey shaking her head.

"Where I'm from, there's no word for 'goodbye,'" Audrey said, standing perfectly still. "Go in peace."

Jane closed the door behind her, leaving Audrey's world and returning to the one she knew. She spotted Crow perched on the fence that separated Audrey's trailer from the neighbor's, head cocked, watching Jane. Jane threw up a hand in a half-wave, feeling as though some sort of acknowledgement was in order but not sure she wanted anyone to see her bidding goodbye to a crow. *No word for goodbye*, Audrey had said. *Well, okay then, au revoir, Crow. Until I see you again.*

She hurried down the path, conscious of the time, when a racket started up in the old cherry tree just outside the gates. She sighed, exasperated. *Can I not get away from crows for just* one *minute?* she thought. As she passed under the tree, two bodies dropped like bombs onto the trail in front of her, then grabbed her, one around the legs, one around the waist, and tackled her to the ground. It was only Amy's snorting laughter and Flory's high-pitched squeal that kept her from thinking she was being ambushed for real. "Nothing . . ." she gasped out as they lay guffawing in the dirt, "like good friends . . . to keep you down to earth!"

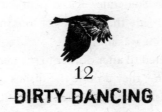

12
DIRTY DANCING

*I*F THAT'S MIKE MACGILLIVRAY *who just walked in, Amy and Flory are going to pay for this with their lives,* Jane decided, her face reflecting the seriousness of her intent. They'd arrived at the dance—the first of the Cultus Lake season—about fifteen minutes ago, and Amy and Flory were already on the crowded dance floor with Ben and Mark, laughing and bouncing happily in time to one of the Cult-Us's new cover tunes. Jane stood in the corner of the Community Hall next to the concession counter, nursing a lukewarm iced tea and wondering how she was supposed to send the right message to anybody covered in dirt and grass stains.

She caught a nod from Mr. Verde up on the stage, an advertising colleague of her mom's and an impressive bass guitarist, and lifted her hand in a little wave. The community's home-grown band was made up of Cultus regulars in their forties and fifties, talented amateur musicians who could pick up any hit and make it their own. She sighed and took another sip of her iced tea. Downright tepid. And a non-biodegradable straw.

Disaster drink. Someone's flared pant leg brushed her shin and she made the mistake of looking down. She sighed again. She was filthy.

They'd waited til after dinner to shower and change, only by the time they'd done the dishes and Amy and Flory had finished their bathroom ablutions, the little cabin had run out of hot water. Jane had wiped off most of the dust and dirt with a cold cloth, and pulled her long, heavy hair, limp from heat and sweat, back and up off her neck. But when her two friends had appeared, sweet-smelling and sparkling in their new dresses, and she remembered she didn't even have her skirt to change into, she'd almost stayed home. In the end, they had literally dragged her down the lane to the Hall, whining and laughing the whole way.

And now Mike MacGillivray was here, and by the looks of him, Katrina D'Angelo couldn't be far behind. He stood in the doorway of the hall, hands gripping the frame on each side, eagerly scanning the room. He wore a loose, white collared shirt, unbuttoned at the neck against the heat, black dress pants, and stylish, square-toed black loafers. Ordinarily an unruly mass of sandy curls, tonight his hair was slicked back off the sides of his face. Against the backdrop of a starry night and bathed in blue and yellow light from the overhead spots, he looked like a picture from a magazine.

Or a character at a masquerade ball, Jane thought. *Even though he's not wearing a mask, it's like I can't tell who he is*. Where was the guy she'd grown up with, the one who went everywhere in a T-shirt and jeans, the one who was going to quit school after this year and become an organic farmer? And why did any of that matter at all to her, anyway?

Several heads turned to stare—female heads, Jane noticed—and she waited for the moment when he would catch sight of the face he was looking for. Then he did. He grinned, and the mask fell away. Crossing the room in a few long strides, he held out his hand: "Dance?"

"Oh! Uh, well, I haven't finished . . ." Jane held up her iced tea, stunned into silence. Mike took the glass from her hand and set it on the counter. Then he took her hand and led her onto the dance floor. Flory glanced over, raising her eyebrows and smiling. Behind Mike's back so that only Jane could see, Amy fluffed a finger under her upturned nose. Jane wasn't sure if it was a comment on her brother's dressy clothes or expensive-smelling cologne, but knowing Amy, figured it could be applied either way. She noted peripherally that the music had not shifted into slow mode when the song changed, and was weak-kneed with gratitude. With an effort of will, she attempted to coordinate the suddenly random and spastic movements of her limbs with the beat of a song she could barely hear over the roaring sound in her ears. *Three minutes*, Jane told herself. *Most songs are only three minutes long. You'll live.*

"You okay?" Mike appeared to have full control of

his own physical functions and was moving in time to the music. It wasn't fair. "You look great, by the way. I really like your hair like that!"

"What?" Jane burst out laughing, and the sensation was like stepping out of a carnival fun house into the light of day. *There* was the real Mike MacGillivray, noticing instantly what a mess she was in her jeans and flip-flops, tank top still sporting a patch of dirt, hair a rat's nest on the top of her head. Kicking her when she was down and dirty, in true boys-against-the-girls style. Now, this was more like it. This she could handle.

"Oh, thanks Mike! I like your hair, too!" she shouted over the music. "Did you use sweat to get it to stick like that? I did! And nice outfit! Whoohee! Maybe we should put in a request with the Cult-Us to play 'Stayin' Alive' for you! You could show us all your *Saturday Night Fever* moves!" She laughed, enjoying her own jokes, and barely registered seeing the smile waver on his face.

"I was at the wildlife center on Thursday," she continued, dancing normally now that she'd finally relaxed, "and I noticed that I'm starting to be able to recognize animals by their scent. You know, like, a skunk's pretty obvious, stinks like burnt rubber, but even a crow has kind of a half-nutty, half-musky odor that's pretty distinct. And a coyote! You ever smell a coyote up close, you'll never forget it. Cross between old sneakers and limberger cheese. Now you . . ." she leaned in close and sniffed, " . . . you smell like, hmmm, an Armani? No, a

Calvin Klein? Wait, don't tell me . . . an Old Spice! Am I right?" She laughed again, but then noticed Mike wasn't laughing with her. He was still moving in time to the music, but his smile was tense, and a small line had appeared between his brows. He was looking at her as though . . . *As though what?* Jane thought. *As though he doesn't recognize me.*

Well, he started the teasing match, she thought. But she decided it might be time to change the subject. "So, you tell your folks yet?" she shouted the question over a song that was demanding a lot of audience participation. "About ditching university for the farming life? I noticed Katrina still seems to be in the dark!"

Mike blushed and looked down, then back up at Jane, the tension in his face intensified and the smile gone. "I've been meaning to, but I'm just not sure if . . ."

"Mike!" she yelled, raising her hands to her head in mock exasperation. "What are you waiting for? You graduate in a *month*!" A troubling thought occurred to her. "Hey, you haven't changed your mind, have you?"

"No, I . . . well, I mean . . . not exactly," Mike stammered, clearly uncomfortable now, "but I've been wondering if there's some way I can . . . do both? Katrina has a point, I mean, about an engineer's salary versus a farmer's, and maybe I can achieve the same . . ."

"I can't believe this!" Jane said, genuinely shocked. So he *had* told Katrina his plan. And she was trying to talk him out of it! Jane wondered suddenly whether

Katrina was aware of the role Jane herself had played in Mike's decision. Her voice went quiet, but she knew Mike was lip-reading every word she said. "Last fall, you tell me you're proud of me for what I'm doing for animals, and how that's helped you decide to take a risk and do something *you* really want to do—instead of what your girlfriend or your parents want you to do." She started shouting again. "And now you're blowing it?" She waved a dismissive hand at him. "For some fancy clothes and, what next, a flashy car?"

"Blowing it?" His eyes went wide with surprise, and something else Jane couldn't read. "I'm not . . . oh, man, I don't *know* what I'm doing!" He was keening from side to side, swaying back and forth in the sea of swirling bodies. Jane planted herself, her hands on her hips, as though challenging him to stand his ground. "I thought I knew . . . but there's someone else in my life to consider, too, you know? If we get married, if we have a family, I have to be sure I can support . . . don't you see, Jane? I have to think ahead. It's not so simple!"

Married? Family? Did he mean with Katrina? Jane didn't see. Couldn't see. The spotlights from the stage seemed suddenly to be glaring directly into her eyes, and the music grated in her ears, overloud, discordant. She let her arms fall to her sides, and her pained disbelief show on her face.

"Hey, you two! What are we missing? Looks dramatic, whatever it is!" Amy had one arm around

Ben's waist and was reapplying her lipgloss with the other hand. "Speaking of which, you're going to catch it, Mike! Aren't you supposed to be picking Katrina up for dinner right about now?"

Mike nodded, not bothering to check his watch. "I . . . I had something on my mind," he answered his sister. "I came here to talk to a friend about it." He looked directly at Jane then. "But I couldn't find her." He turned and walked out of the hall without looking back.

"Whoa." Amy looked up at Jane, eyebrows raised, waiting for an explanation. Jane stood, arms stiff at her sides, staring at the empty doorway of the Cultus Lake Community Hall. So he hadn't been teasing her after all. He'd *meant* his compliments. She realized with a sick sense of shame that she hadn't been teasing either. She'd meant her insults. He'd come to her looking for a sounding board as he waded through a decision that could cost him dearly—the approval of his family, his relationship with Katrina—and what had she done? *What had she done?*

"I've got to go," she choked out. She took off at a run.

13
THE LAST FLIGHT OF CORVUS

*T*HOSE WHO NEED HER MEDICINE *will find her at crossroads . . .*

Audrey's words echoed in Jane's head, her feet pounding their rhythm into the dirt of the forest floor. She ran hard, panting for breath and not caring, wanting only to put distance between herself and the dance hall, between herself and herself. *What kind of friend . . . ? What kind of person . . . ?*

Was that what crow medicine was all about? If so, she wanted none of it.

She ran until the strains of music and laughter behind her faded and disappeared, and the glow from the lanterns hanging around the outside of the hall was replaced by starglow and moonlight. When the only sounds she could hear were her own breathing and the crunch of dry twigs and pine needles, she slowed, letting her eyes adjust to the myriad shades of night-time in the woods.

There, just ahead and to her right, was the path to the lakeshore trail, and the way back to the MacGillivray cabin. On her left, just up ahead, was the path to the village shops, to Logan's. Before her, the trail branched off several times, leading to this or that laneway of cabins. And behind her lay the way back to the Community Hall. No through road—no way was she going back *there*. And she didn't feel like going home to bed yet. It was too dark for a lakeside walk, too late to hang out at the shops, too early in the long weekend to get in her car and make the hour-long drive back to Cedar's Ridge. Which is exactly what she felt like doing.

A tiny orange glow winked suddenly in the periphery of her vision, and almost simultaneously she caught the scent of woodsmoke on the air. The fire. She'd forgotten there would be a bonfire tonight. "Maybe you'll make it to the fire," Audrey had said. *Yeah, well, so maybe you were right about one stupid thing, Audrey.*

A minute later, Jane emerged into the little clearing, dirty, sweaty, and panting, to choruses of "Make room for another guest!" and "Put another S'more on the fire for the newcomer!" No one asked her why she wasn't at the dance, and she was thankful not to have to explain. Marg and Malcolm MacGillivray were there, playing cards by firelight with the DiSalvos from the cabin next door. Mr. and Mrs. Nazarali from Driftwood Street were there with their two little twin girls, who were singing songs together quietly as they watched marshmallow after marshmallow catch fire and fall into the flames. "They don't like the taste of them," Mrs. Nazarali explained with a smile, seeing Jane stare. "But they love to roast things over a campfire, don't you, girls?"

Audrey was not there. Well, maybe poker had gotten serious. Jane felt a hysterical giggle bubble up as she thought, *Maybe they've branched out into strip poker.* She had a sudden flash of Eunice seductively sliding one of those pink plastic curlers out of her hair and throwing it to the floor each time she lost a hand, and almost laughed out loud. "I think I will have a S'more, Mr. DiSalvo, if you don't mind," she said, seating herself on a log between the two groups and helping herself to graham crackers and chocolate chips. For a moment, the only sounds in the clearing were the crackling of the fire and the shuffling of cards.

"We were just talking about the stars, Jane," Mr. DiSalvo spoke to her as he dealt another round. "Trying to see how many constellations we could spot with the naked eye, and how many we actually knew the names of. Riaz here is quite the astronomer!"

"Good night for it," Jane agreed, gazing up through the circle of tall trees that surrounded them. She found the North Star, and made out Ursa Major and Ursa Minor easily—the Big and Little Dippers.

"It was the Greeks, of course, who called it Ursa Major—the Great Bear," said Riaz Nazarali, following her gaze and carving shapes out of the sky with his hand. "But the Brits called it a plough, the French a saucepan. The Chinese decided it was a celestial chariot for one of the sky deities, and in the Hindu tradition it is called the Seven Rishis—the Wise Men." He paused to put two small foil packets into the coals for his daughters. "Several North American Aboriginal tribes, including the Mi'kmaq of Canada's east coast, see the bowl of the Big Dipper as a bear, and the stars of the handle as the hunters who are tracking him. In the 1800s, runaway slaves followed what they called 'the drinking gourd' to the northern states. And so to them, that constellation was a symbol of freedom."

"Are there any other star animals, papa?" asked one of the twins as she wiped charred marshmallow onto her pants with a surreptitious glance at her mom.

"Officially," he replied, "the night sky is home to fourteen people, nine birds, two insects, nineteen land animals, ten water creatures, two centaurs, one head of hair, a serpent, a dragon, a flying horse, a river, and twenty-nine inanimate objects. That we know of. So, yes, Melia. Many others. Excellent question."

"Wow," Jane breathed. "You really do know your stars!" Thinking of all the times she'd looked up at the night sky from her bedroom window at home, or from the front deck in summer, always in wonder but also mostly in ignorance, she marveled at how much there was to be known. She pointed to a trapezium shape just to the north of Virgo, the maiden, which she knew from astrology. "Any idea what that one is?" She knew Aquila, the eagle, and Leo Minor, the little lion, and Orion, the hunter, and it wasn't any of those.

"Ah, yes!" Mr. Nazarali nodded in excitement, seemingly pleased with her discovery. He pulled the two hot packets from the fire and set their sweet, gooey contents out for Maya and Melia before returning his attention to the sky. "Eleven stars visible to the naked eye, including Alchiba, Gienah Ghurab, Algorab, Minkar, and Kraz, the last of these a staggering two hundred and ninety light years away. This constellation will disappear from the northern hemisphere after May, and will not appear again until January. Well done, Jane. You've caught the last flight of Corvus—the Crow."

For a moment, Jane sat in stunned silence, then she groaned in disbelief. And then she started to laugh. Surrounded. She was surrounded by crows. Inundated. Infiltrated. Inhabited. *You already have it, Jane—crow medicine*. It was inside her. One of her mother's favorite sayings flashed through her mind: "Wherever you go, there you are." She glanced skyward again. Yes, there was Corvus, directly overhead. Over her head. Wherever she went, there, too, would go Crow.

Sensing particular interest in his audience, Mr. Nazarali launched into the story of Corvus. "The Greek god Apollo sent the crow out with a goblet to collect water," he began, pitching his voice low as though he were recounting a ghost story. "But the independent-minded creature neglected to do the job he'd been assigned and spent his afternoon feasting on delicious figs instead.

Wouldn't you?" His little girls giggled. "When the hour came to return to Apollo, the crow realized he would have to explain how he had used up all his time and still not managed to come back with the water. Spotting a water snake, he seized it in his claws and flew back to Apollo, explaining when he arrived that this writhing creature was the reason for his failure. Realizing at once that the crow was trying to trick him, Apollo threw all three—the crow, the goblet, and the water snake—into the heavens." Here, Mr. Nazarali paused and pointed out Crater and Hydra in the sky above their fire, to the north and west of Corvus. "As for the crow, in punishment for having failed to return with the water, he was made to suffer eternal thirst. Which is why the crow caahs as he does instead of singing beautifully like all the other birds!"

The DiSalvos and the MacGillivrays set down their cards and clapped. "Bravo, Riaz!" "Brilliantly told!" "Cheers!" This last was shouted by the men over the clinking of beer bottles.

"I have a crow story, too, come to think of it!" exclaimed Mrs. MacGillivray, abandoning her cards altogether and taking up her mug of hot cocoa. Jane found herself grinning helplessly and shaking her head, resigned to her fate. She could predict with near certainty that Mrs. MacGillivray's crow story would not be the last that night.

"So, do you all know the legend of the Phoenix?"

Mrs. MacGillivray asked, looking slowly around the circle. Maya and Melia, their eyes wide and sparkling in the firelight and their mouths ringed with chocolate, shook their heads in unison. "Well, you see, the Phoenix is a magical bird that lives for a thousand years. And at the end of that thousand years, it builds a funeral pyre and throws itself into the flames and dies." The twins gasped in horror. "But!" Mrs. MacGillivray held up a hand. "As the fire dies down, the Phoenix—or the Firebird, as some call it—is born anew, and rises from the ashes on wings of flame to live for another thousand years."

The little girls clapped their hands and cried, "Yaaaayyy!"

Jane frowned. "I thought you said you had a crow story, Mrs. M."

"Well!" she answered. "That's the interesting thing! There are a number of theories as to how the Phoenix legend came about. One is that someone saw a peacock backlit by the setting sun and believed the bird was on fire. But another theory is that it was a crow! Now, a crow does something called 'anting,' where it'll disturb an ants' nest, spread its wings, and let the ants swarm its body. The ants give the crow a full-body massage, and at the same time, they feast on these bugs called feather mites that live on the crow and drive him crazy. A win-win, as they say. Sometimes, though, the crow will sit himself over a hot surface instead, such as the dying embers of a fire, to get rid of the mites and enjoy a bit of a sauna. When he's ready to fly away and begins to flap his wings, the rush of air may be enough to rouse the fire to life again. And so what you see . . ."

"Is a Firebird rising from the ashes!" Mr. MacGillivray finished, intrigued by his wife's story. "Where did you learn all that, hon? Not TSN, I'm thinking!"

Mr. DiSalvo laughed. Mrs. MacGillivray made a face. "One of those science channels, I think," she replied.

Not to be outdone, Mr. MacGillivray cleared his throat and announced that he would now regale them with an ancient Scottish poem about crows that he had learned as a boy. Jane glanced at Mrs. MacGillivray, who was rolling her eyes exactly like Amy, and giggled. The rest of the family was always mildly embarrassed by Mr. M's shows of Scottish nostalgia, but Jane thrilled to the sound of his broad brogue and over-the-top theatricality.

"The Twa Corbies," he began, clearing his throat once again as he shook out his shoulders and tilted his head to either side to stretch his neck. He lowered his voice and began:

"As I was walking all alane,
I heard twa corbies making a mane;
The tane unto the t'other say,
'Where sall we gang and dine today?'
In behint yon auld fail dyke,

I wot there lies a new slain knight;
And naebody kens that he lies there,
But his hawk, his hound, and lady fair.
His hound is to the hunting gane,
His hawk to fetch the wild-fowl hame,
His lady's ta'en another mate,
So we may mak our dinner sweet.
Ye'll sit on his white hause-bane,
And I'll pike out his bonny blue een;
Wi'ae lock o' his gowden hair
We'll theek our nest when it grows bare.
Mony a one for him makes mane,
But nane sall ken where he is gane;
O'er his white banes, when they are bare,
The wind sall blaw for evermair."

There was silence, and then: "For the love of all
things holy, Malcolm, you've frightened the wee girls
half to death!" Mrs. MacGillivray reached over and
punched her husband's shoulder, only half-playfully,
clearly spooked herself. The twins, Jane noticed, hadn't
actually understood enough of Mr. M's accent to feel
anything one way or the other, but she shivered herself
as a tremor ran the length of her spine.

"You are reminding me, Malcolm," Mrs. Nazarali
spoke now, quietly. "Something is going on with one of
the cabins on Driftwood Street. Strange things. People
are saying it is haunted." She laughed nervously. "Silly,

really. There is no such thing, right? But strange noises at night, lights going on and off, people say. I've seen things, too. Always at night. And yet it is empty, all boarded up. It has been that way since last fall."

"Which one is it, Fahrza?" Mrs. DiSalvo asked. Jane noticed she crossed herself the way Flory often did.

Driftwood Street, she thought, something tugging at her memory. *Wasn't that where . . .*

"The one with all the garden ornaments, you know? And the bright red door. I am sorry to say I never found those people very congenial. What was their name, honey? Oh, wait now, I remember . . . the Harbinsales."

Jane had retrieved her charred S'more from the coals and was attempting to eat the less black bits, but now it slipped from her grasp and dropped, foil and all, into the flames. Mr. MacGillivray chose that moment to throw a handful of spruce boughs onto the fire, and when the smoke finally cleared, there, just outside the circle, stood Audrey.

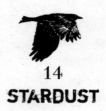

14
STARDUST

"**G**OT ANY OF THAT SAGE WITH YOU TONIGHT, Audrey?" Mr. MacGillivray asked, yawning and stretching and using the excuse to put his arm around his wife. "I always have the best dreams after one of your sage fires."

"Matter of fact, I do," she answered, reaching into one of the pockets of her faded Macintosh.

Audrey had joined the circle, and the conversation had turned abruptly from the ostensible haunting of the Harbinsale cabin to more mundane matters: Mr. Logan's new security mirrors and burgeoning selection of organic produce, which cabins were up for sale this spring, how Audrey was getting along with the new managers at the trailer park. Seemed everybody knew Audrey, *and* her real name. Had it only been Jane, Amy, and Flory who'd thought of her as the Crone all these years? Jane blushed at the thought, ashamed and glad of the darkness.

Audrey pulled out a small cloth pouch and worked at the drawstring until she could fit her hand inside.

Withdrawing a mound of dry, whitish-green leaves, she said, "Jane was just asking me about dreaming this afternoon, that right, Jane?" Her eyes crinkled at the corners as she smiled. Reaching forward, she sprinkled the dried sage over the flames.

Jane nodded, sleepy. Covering a yawn with her hand, she closed her eyes and breathed in the sweet smoky smell of burning sage. The voices of the others receded into the distance and the crackling of the fire grew closer, until it was the only thing she could hear.

Dry twigs, snapping like small bones. Dessicated pine needles, cracking in half and releasing their faint resiny scent to her nostrils. The near-silent parting of tall grasses as something passed through them. Soundlessly, she crept over the knoll, following the tiny creature ahead of her, its footfalls almost inaudible in the rustling blades. The creature paused, and so she paused, too, catching sight as she did so of her own reflection in the creek that fed the lake. Magnificent white, almost glowing in the light of the noon sun. Ears white, pale pink inside, pale pink nose, white whiskers—she swished her tail and watched it dance above her head—all white. She dipped her right front paw into the creek—the black paw—and leaned in to drink the water caught between her paw pads. Right eye blue, left eye green. The sight no longer startled her. There was a time when she'd thought of herself as marked, deformed. Now, she knew she was beautiful.

The creature was on the move again. She crouched

low, ears and nose twitching as she refocused her senses on its scent and sounds. Roasted corn and salt—that's what a mouse smells like.

She took a moment, less than a second, to glance up from the string-thin trail she was following and caught sight of the ancient pine, maybe fifty lengths ahead, the ends of its roots already rippling the ground beneath her paws, the point of its head scraping still, blue sky. The tree was the mouse's destination, she knew, and it was her task to ensure her charge arrived alive.

Every instinct in her was tracking the mouse, stalking, hunting, making ready to seize her prey. She felt a familiar ache in her jaw, and a droplet of saliva slid down her canine tooth and fell to the dry earth below. But something beyond instinct was guiding this journey, and she knew that at its end, she would come away without a meal. Today, her task was different. Food would have to wait.

Less than ten lengths from the base of the tree, she felt the still air above her stir almost imperceptibly. She froze. Without looking up, she knew what moved the winds: it was the red-tail.

Splitting her focus, her senses were trained now on both predator and prey. Had the mouse noticed the hawk? She wasn't sure; the soft, scratching footfalls had not changed their pace. But the hawk, certainly, had spotted the mouse. The shadow that spiraled in the field just ahead and to her right was small, but growing larger by the second. Her instincts measured spirals against foot-falls against distance to the tree, calculations completed faster than thought, and she knew the mouse would not make it. Should she yowl out a warning? Frighten the mouse into increasing its pace? But what if she shocked it, instead, into changing its course? Or para-lyzed it with fear?

The lazy spirals had stopped. Once more, the air was dead still. Then the grasses, too, fell silent. She realized the mouse knew. The rest of its life was measured in seconds. Swifter than stone, the hawk fell, wings held tight to its sides, and she watched as the shadow grew like ripples on a lake, larger, larger . . .

She pounced. Snaring the mouse between her two front paws, claws carefully retracted, she buried it beneath her. She heard a terrible screech that sounded of fury and pain, and realized it was her own voice that cried as inch-long talons sank into the skin of her back and buried themselves in her flesh. Like a jet engine reversing its engines upon landing, the hawk halted its downward trajectory and reoriented every muscle and feather for takeoff. She felt her skin tear as the hawk lifted her with him, half an inch, then an inch, then two inches off the ground, the air around her churning with the fury of his wings. Still she held the mouse between her paws.

And then suddenly she was free. Unable to bear her weight, the hawk had withdrawn his talons and shot thirty feet into the air. He circled, waiting for another chance. She had time to be grateful that her attacker had not been an eagle—she was small—and to wonder whether her own attack had frightened the mouse to death, before she saw it scurry free, making straight for the tree. This time, she matched its pace, keeping her body between it and the hawk, never giving the raptor his second chance. As they came level with the tree, she glanced left in time to see the mouse propel itself into a small opening at its base and disappear.

Down, down, down, twists this way, turns that way, and around and around and out. Into the burrow. Home. Small things. All mine. I see, I smell, I feel, I hear, I know everything here. In place. In order. Home. Mine. Safe.

She was with the mouse in a dark, cavernous opening beneath the tree that smelled of earth and rainwater and was alive with the movements of worms and small insects and the living roots of the tree above. She was aware of its thoughts, and seemed not to see but to sense, to follow the mouse with her mind as it checked on its stores of seeds, as it ate to replenish the energy it had spent in its perilous journey across the field, as it rested its heart, knowing it was safe and alive, at least for now.

She waited—for a sign, a word, an explanation. Why here? Why a mouse? The cat she had understood. The cat was strong and agile, intelligent, fierce when necessary. A fighter. A worthy ally. But a mouse? A mouse was weak, everybody's prey. A mouse was so small.

What little light had illumined the cavern suddenly

disappeared and her vision went black. A flash of hot terror shot through her as she realized she was trapped under the ground, vulnerable to attack from any of the tunnels that led to the burrow, with nothing but a mouse to help her. Opening her eyes wider and straining to perceive something, anything, in the void, she thought she saw a flicker of something very close to her face. She caught her breath, her heart hammering like a war drum in her own ears. The eye took shape in the darkness, a shining orb of deep brown that was larger than the size of her entire head. Then she saw the nose below it, long, pink-tipped, short hairs bristling and whiskers quivering, so close to her own that nothing more than a sheet of onionskin could have passed between the two of them. She and the mouse. For it was the mouse.

It spoke as though from inside her own head: I AM NOT SMALL. She fought the urge to laugh, half-hysterical with fear and surprise. My spirit is not small. Remember this. But I help you see the small, so that you may know those whom you protect.

The vision faded, and she found herself in a tunnel outside the burrow, not the one by which she'd arrived, but one she knew would lead her out again. Half walking, half gliding, she made her way through the dirt passage, circling upward, climbing back toward the surface of the earth. The soil grew lighter, less dense, light flooded the tunnel, and she knew she was nearly there. Hurrying now, she sped by the little bedchamber and had to double back *to check whether her eyes had deceived her. They had not. Tucked cozily into bed, blankets drawn up around her chin, nightcap and reading glasses in place and a book of faerie tales in her tiny hands, the mouse glanced up from her reading, gave her a wink and a wave, then turned back to her book, giggling like a delighted grandmother. Shaking her head in wonder, she turned to complete her journey to the surface and found she was already there.*

The tunnel had deposited her beneath the deck of her own house, and she had to hop forward from rock to stone to grass to get clear of the overhang before she could take flight. And then she was in the air. Overjoyed, she climbed hard and fast til she caught a slight eddy in the balmy air, and then she spread her wings to their full span and glided out over the lake. Oh, the lake! The crooked circle of it somehow the shape of her own life— imperfect, beautiful, whole. Blue and sheened with silver sunlight, it sparkled like a treasure she might like to line her nest with, and she fought the instinct to swoop down and try to tear a piece free. She crowed instead because, well, somebody had to say something, and listened to the answering calls from each of the four corners. Yes, it was a good day. Even the old red-tail turned for the woods when it saw the glint in her eye. Oh, yes. It was a very good day.

Jane's head fell forward and her chin hit her chest, startling her awake. She took in a deep breath of midnight air scented with woodsmoke and looked around, blinking. Mrs. Nazarali held sleeping twins in her lap, and rested her own head on her husband's shoulder. Mr. MacGillivray lay stretched out on a log, snoring, and Mrs. MacGillivray was slowly packing playing cards, thermoses, and tin foil into her bag. The DiSalvos snuggled side by side, their heads touching, talking quietly. Audrey sat beside her, eyes closed as if she, too, were asleep.

"How long have I been gone?" Jane whispered to herself as she scrubbed her hands over her face.

"Gone?" Audrey was wide awake, it seemed, though her eyes remained closed. "You never left. Maybe fell asleep for a minute there, though." She paused. "Any dreams?"

Hesitating at first, then gathering speed as her tale progressed, Jane told Audrey about the feral cat, the mouse, and the crow. "It was as if part of me was here, awake, still listening to the fire," Jane tried to explain, "and some other part of me was back at Elfin Lake, dreaming. And sometimes I was watching the animals, but sometimes I *was* them!"

"Because you have their medicine," Audrey said. It was a statement, rather than a question. Then she laughed. "I make a pretty convincing hawk, don't you think?"

Jane started. She'd actually forgotten to mention the red-tail. "How did you know about the . . . ?" She shook her head then, hard, trying to clear away the answer that had come to her, the only answer that added up: Audrey had been dreaming with her—had, in fact, been *in* her dream. She looked up at Audrey. The older woman met her eyes, smiling, and nodded.

Jane's understanding of "normal" had been pushed to its limits by the events of the past three days, and this last revelation was enough to make her wonder whether she'd ever think the same way again. Too much more of this and there'd be little kids spying on her from the tops of fruit trees and calling her crazy. She giggled, and giggling made her recall the tittering storybook mouse of her dream.

"Audrey, the mouse told me I was a protector of those who are small," she said, realizing that what was passing for ordinary conversation between the two of them would sound more than a little strange to anyone who might happen to be listening.

Audrey nodded. "The mouse is protector of the small, keeper of the natural order of things, the one who sets things right when they've gone all topsy turvy. Mouse can see what's right in front of her nose, even things other people prefer not to see, and take appropriate action."

Something in Audrey's tone prompted Jane to recall her conversation with Mike. In her mind's eye, she saw herself yelling at him over top of the music and winced. "I could have used some mouse medicine earlier tonight," she said bitterly.

"It's good to know when to use what," Audrey agreed with a sympathetic smile, as though she understood without Jane's having to explain. "Crow medicine can taste bitter goin' down. Mouse medicine is like sugar on the spoon. And the cat—now, Cat will put her own life on the line for her little ones."

"But Audrey," Jane countered, "the mouse wasn't her little one!"

"All the little ones are my little ones," Audrey said, "and all the little ones are your little ones. We're all the same, you know. Stardust. We're all just stardust. All made of the same stuff. Me and the crows. You and the mice. You and me. You and those two mischief-makers!"

Jane turned to find Amy and Flory ambling up the path behind her, still smelling faintly of perfume and raspberry punch. Both were yawning.

"Home, Jane?" Amy inquired, nodding acknow-ledgement to Audrey.

Jane said her goodbyes around the fire, and then she and her friends walked the trail back to the cabin arm in arm, Amy on her left and Flory on her right, each girl lost in her own thoughts. That night, Amy and Flory would dream of dancing, and Jane would dream of the small ones—the hunted, the endangered, the captured, the lost—and wonder what on earth one small mouse could do to save them.

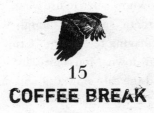

15

COFFEE BREAK

JUST BEYOND THE LAST CURVE in the road, someone was singing. The clear notes floated up over the salmonberry bushes and through the oak trees to mingle with birdsong and the hum of industrious insects already earning their day's keep. The old road was dusty and cracked—the last rainfall had been weeks ago—and the deep ditches held little water. It was almost June, and every green leaf, every nesting bird, the warm, shimmering air itself, held the promise of summer.

Jane rounded the curve, wiping the sweat from her face for the hundredth time since setting out for the wildlife center on foot, and caught sight of Anthony on the Care Center's tiny porch, coffee in one hand and portable phone in the other, singing. And dancing. Between spins, he was gazing up into the old apple tree at the center of the habitat garden, clearly tracking something. Jane took a few more tentative steps, not wanting to interrupt the performance but very eager to hear the words of the song. Anthony worked a wave and a nod into his choreography; so he knew she was there. As far as he was concerned, though, an audience was gold. Jane grinned and hurried forward to join him on the porch. Turning, she followed his gaze until she spotted the robin flitting in and out of the apple tree's gnarled branches, pulling twigs from secret sources all over the garden to build her nest. Anthony sang quietly, underscoring the scene. Jane recognized the tune, but the lyrics were all his own.

"American robin, stay away from me-hee, American robin, birdie let me be-hee." Anthony gestured vehemently with his coffee. Jane gave him a wide berth. "Don't come a peckin' 'round my door, I don't wanna see your beak no more. I got more important things to do than spend my time buildin' nests with you. Now robin, I said stay away-hay. American robin, listen what I say-ay-ay-ay-ay-ay . . ." Winding up with a double jazz pirouette, he landed in the splits on the porch floor, spilling only a minimum of coffee and holding the phone receiver aloft like a baton.

Jane gazed down at him: "Getting back to nature, hey, Anthony?"

"Morning, Jane girl," he replied, downing a slug of coffee. "Go see Evie. She needs a hug." The phone rang in his extended hand. "Good morning, Urban Wildlife Rescue! How may I be of assistance today?"

Inside, Jane found the senior staffer drawing up meds in the exam room. Evie's face looked strained, but she smiled when she saw Jane. "Hey, there!" she called.

"You'll be pleased to know your rescue of last week is doing well and has been added to the regular fledge rounds." Jane made pompoms with her fists and gave a silent cheer, which Evie returned. She started down the hallway toward the kitchen, when suddenly she remembered the question she'd been holding onto all week long.

"Evie, I keep meaning to ask you about those oiled starlings we had last week," she said. "What happened to them? Was there another oil spill?"

Evie shook her head, her face tightening with tension again. "StickiStep," she answered. Jane gave her a blank look. "It's a 'pest control' product anybody can buy and put in their eaves or on their roof if they've got 'pests.'" Evie was making quotation marks with her fingers to indicate exactly what she thought of the term "pest." "The theory is, the birds or mice or squirrels will get the sticky stuff all over their feet and hate it so much it'll deter them from coming back to your house. Reality is, they often get stuck and thrash around trying to get free, which completely coats them in the adhesive. The lucky ones end up here, where we have to cover them in mineral oil to get the adhesive off, then give them an oil spill bath to get the oil off. And you'll remember how *that* process affects their odds for survival."

Jane shuddered, recalling the palpable panic of oiled birds whose only hope of survival was also the most stressful event of their lives—to be held captive by humans and subjected to a bathing and rinsing process that could last up to half an hour. For a wildlife rehabilitator to have to put an animal through that ordeal deliberately, because of somebody else's idea of effective pest control, was almost beyond her ability to comprehend.

"You said the lucky ones?" Jane queried, more than a little afraid of what Evie might say next.

The senior rehabilitator made a noise of disgust. "People cover their eaves in the stuff and then forget to check it. Animals starve to death, trapped in StickiStep, unable to get to food or water. Or sometimes a predator puts them out of their misery before that happens. After all, they're easy pickings." Her eyes sad, she shook her head, as though trying to erase some of the memories it held. "Somebody brought us a mouse once, stuck to the stuff and near dead of starvation or dehydration, couldn't tell which, patches of skin and hair missing where the glue had ripped it off, one of its front legs severed where it had chewed it off in an attempt to escape. I put him down." She drew a deep breath. "There are so many humane ways for people to keep their homes free of wild animals. I don't know how this stuff can still be legal."

Impulsively, Jane stepped forward and put her arms around her. "Anthony said you needed a hug," she murmured.

"Oh!" Evie hugged Jane hard in return, then stepped back. "Yeah." She laughed a little. "Well, I don't think it was oiled starlings he had in mind, actually." Clearing her throat, she said, "Would you ask the rest of the morning crew to spare me a few minutes at the end of your coffee break? I've got some . . . some news." With that, she turned back to the syringes and feeding tubes that lay on the exam room counter, and Jane made her way to the kitchen to start diets for the fledgling birds.

The Care Center was bursting with new life. Every square inch of space was piled high with it, cage upon basket upon kennel upon aviary, and the warm air in the care room was sharp and bright with the insistent calls of hungry young—starlings, jays, chickadees, robins, thrushes, crows. Beth hurried between the kitchen and the isolation room, where literally buckets of nestlings raised their gaping mouths to her constantly for food. Frank, Katrina, and Avis kept the outside doors swinging on their hinges as they cleaned and fed the birds in the songbird aviary, the duck pens, the swan pen, the raptor pen, and six duckling brooders. Thirty-eight mallard ducklings in all this morning, handfuls of down and energy, nowhere near able to fly but with legs seemingly made of springs that could catapult them out of your hands and right out the door if you weren't on your guard.

"Coffee!" Avis sang as she brushed past Jane on her way to reception. Jane swung around to stare at the clock: 11:20. How was it possible? "Mind you come, missy. This might be our last chance before summer swings into high gear." Jane laughed in disbelief. *This wasn't high gear?* Just how many more animals could they fit in here? She finished the round, set her timer, and slipped it into her pocket. Then she followed Avis to the basement of the house on the far side of the garden.

The 1920s-era house had once been someone's home, but now served as the administration offices for the Urban Wildlife Rescue Center. Downstairs, the room that looked out onto the back garden had been turned into a lunchroom for the volunteers, and there Jane found Avis pouring coffee into two ice-filled tumblers and setting out a plate of ginger-chocolate-chunk cookies.

"Wow, Avis!" Jane exclaimed. "Nice treat—thanks!"

"It's no treat," Avis responded crossly. "It's a necessity! This heat is going to kill me. And it's not even summer yet! I don't know how I'm going to manage. I'm no spring chicken any more, you know." She took a long draught of the iced coffee and closed her eyes, sighing heavily.

Jane looked closely at her friend. The older woman had once seemed ancient to her, but as they'd gotten to know one another, Jane had come to think of her as just Avis. She had forgotten that Avis was older, and that the hard physical work the Center required was likely even harder for her. As the patient load increased and the temperature rose, Jane could see that the next few months could become a real challenge. She wondered if there were any way she could finish her fledge rounds faster in order to help Avis with the outside pens.

"Now tell me, how was your long weekend, missy?" Avis interrupted her thoughts. "Meet any nice young men at the dance?"

Jane groaned, her worries about her friend momentarily forgotten. "You won't even believe it when I tell you, Avis." Jane recounted the events of the previous weekend, starting with the afternoon at the Shack with Amy and Flory and ending with her dream by the fire at Cultus. "Now that I'm back in the city doing homework and coming here and everything seems normal again, I can almost pretend all that stuff didn't happen. But that's the thing, Avis—*it did*. It's like there's Audrey's world and then there's the real world—my world—but now there's this line where they overlap, and somehow I stepped across that line! I mean, it all seemed to make sense at the time, what she said about Crow, my dream about the animals." She paused, searching for words. "I know those things aren't real, of course. But Avis, *they felt like they were!*" She looked at her friend, eyes wide with surprise at her own admission.

Avis looked at her thoughtfully and took her time before replying. "I'm a practical woman, Jane, as you know," she said finally. "All my life, I've believed only in the things I could see with my own eyes and touch with my own two hands. But let me tell you, when my first husband died, I wanted more than anything in the world to believe there was something more, something beyond what my senses told me was real. I'll never forget that longing. It might just be the strongest thing I've ever felt."

Jane was grateful her friend hadn't laughed at her strange story, had, in fact, actually understood her. She had a sudden thought: "Avis, after your husband died, did you ever feel, or dream, or maybe sense . . . ?" Jane was saved the trouble of finding the right words. Avis cut her off.

"No, I did not." She stood abruptly and busied herself with the dishes in the sink. Jane played with the crumbs on her plate, wondering if she ought to say something more, when Avis spoke again. "But that's not to say I don't believe it might be possible for others. For you, maybe."

"What's possible for Jane?" Katrina chimed as she breezed in, cheeks rosy with heat and exertion, blond hair flying. "To still find a boyfriend for the summer? Don't worry, sweetie, it'll happen! I believe there's a perfect guy for every girl. Me and Mike are proof of that. Any cookies left, Avis?"

"In my backpack," Avis replied. "And I was just saying to Jane there's no reason why she couldn't date *both* the young fellows who asked her out this weekend. Wouldn't you agree, Katrina?"

Jane turned her guffaw into a cough just as Beth and Frank walked in together. Speaking of romance, something else had clearly transpired between last Thursday and this! The two summer staffers weren't holding hands or even looking at each other. But their faces were smiling the same smile. *Well, isn't spring just bustin' out all over and whoopity doo-da,* Jane thought, feeling like a miserly old curmudgeon. But then again, she had her two imaginary boyfriends to keep her company. She was grinning again over Avis's fantastic lie when Evie arrived.

"I'll get right to the point," the senior rehabilitator said, tossing her clipboard down on the kitchen table. She remained standing as the members of the Thursday morning crew gathered around her, curiosity aroused. "You are all aware of the progression of West Nile Virus across the North American continent. And anybody with ears and a television set has heard the predictions that it will arrive in British Columbia this summer, most likely via the Fraser Valley. Mosquitoes are the vectors and birds are the carriers, with corvids most drastically affected, and crows most susceptible of all. There is no specific medication and no cure, only supportive care, and the prognosis for corvids is universally poor." Although none of this information was new, Jane felt her heart beat faster at Evie's mention of crows.

"Until recently," Evie continued, "we had no evidence that bird-to-bird transmission was possible, which meant that running a close-quarters facility like the UWRC, where quarantine is not possible, and caring for over two thousand patients during mosquito season alone, was still an option." She cleared her throat, the only sign that what she was saying was a struggle. "Although we still don't know whether birds can pass the virus to other birds in the wild, we now know that it can be transmitted bird to bird in confined settings. Such as here."

Frank raised his hand. "In a minute," Evie shook her head. "Let me finish." She looked around at each member of the team. "It may not have occurred to you before that although our primary mandate here is to care for animals, our first responsibility is to *you*. Your health, your safety." Jane still could not see where Evie was going with this line of reasoning, but she was beginning to understand why the young woman's face held the cares and concerns of someone much older.

"It was once thought bird-to-bird transmission was not possible," Evie repeated. "We now know it is. It's still believed that bird-to-human transmission is not possible. But we could find out tomorrow—or in October, after weeks and weeks of repeated exposure— that it is. And that's a risk the staff here are not willing to take. Frank, I said in a minute, please."

She took a deep breath. "The staff have made a formal recommendation to the UWRC board of directors for the adoption of a new policy that we think is our best hope for protecting both the majority of animals in our care as well as the staff and volunteers who work here.

After a very difficult vote, which split the board, the motion was passed." Jane glanced up in surprise as she heard Evie's voice waver. "Starting first thing Monday morning and until the end of September—the end of mosquito season—we will be euthanizing all crows admitted to the UWRC."

16

SHOOT THE MESSENGER

J ANE'S HAND FLEW TO HER HEART. *No*, she wanted to say. *No, that was just a dream. Not real.* But Evie's calm, rational voice continued on.

"We hope that we can counsel as many members of the public as possible to leave nestlings and fledglings alone, to refrain from bringing them here unless they are absolutely sure those birds have been abandoned or orphaned," she said. "Jane, that will be an important part of your job as part of the mobile rescue team. We get so many UHI animals in the summer—unnecessary human intervention," she explained. "Anyway, until we can know a hundred percent for sure that humans are safe in the same close quarters with WNV crows, or until such time as we receive a mega-dollar donation to conduct laboratory diagnostics or build a quarantine facility, our policy will be as I have stated. Are there any questions? Frank?"

"Yes, uh, with all due respect, Evie, there's a vaccine, you know." Frank gazed up at his supervisor, smiling benignly. Jane wondered whether he could possibly have intended his words to pack as much of a slap as they had.

"Yes, as a matter of fact, I do know, Frank," Evie replied calmly. "A vaccine was developed in 2002 for horses, who are also very susceptible to WNV and who are of course very valuable to their owners. Which is presumably why research money was allocated to them first. Preliminary vaccines for birds became available in 2004 and 2005, but they're still in the experimental stages, and what's more, the treatment costs over fifty dollars per animal. We get two thousand animals in here during mosquito season, Frank, most of them birds. You do the math." Evie took a deep breath and looked up at the ceiling, then closed her eyes and slowly blew the air out of her lungs. She was fighting for control, Jane could see, and the very idea frightened her. Evie was always in control. Jane counted on it. They all did.

"Any other questions?" Evie asked, opening her eyes. The little kitchen was silent, save for the hum of the old refrigerator. Evie nodded. "Well, if you think of any later on, don't hesitate to ask. Oh, I should let you know . . . several members of the board quit over this decision, and we've already lost several volunteers as well. No staff so far." She carefully avoided looking at Frank. "It's understandable that people will have strong feelings, one way or the other, and I appreciate how important it is to act according to what you believe to be right. So if you feel you can't support this decision, I will regretfully accept your resignation, but you will have my understanding and there will be no hard feelings."

Evie took up her clipboard from the table and headed for the door, then turned back. "Jane, come see me after your coffee break, would you?" She left without waiting for an answer.

The lunchroom erupted as the door closed behind her. "This is horrible!" Katrina exclaimed, tossing her hair for emphasis. "How can they ask us to go along with it?"

"Are you crazy?" Beth challenged her. "You do understand that people can die from this thing, don't you? Face it, Kat, they're doing the right thing, protecting the staff and volunteers. They couldn't run this place without us!"

"Couldn't afford the lawsuit, either, I suppose, if one of us died." Avis spoke quietly, so that only Jane caught her words.

Katrina shook her head. "I don't know, you guys. I mean, what are you going to do if you find an injured crow this summer? One you know could get better? Are you going to bring it here, knowing it'll be euthanized?" Jane thought again of the little fledge she'd rescued the week before. And of her dream. *All the crows will have to die.*

"Frank," Beth implored, sounding uncertain now, "you're on side, right?"

"Oh, absolutely, Beth," Frank echoed, that agreeable

smile back on his face. The Center has a duty to protect its key resource. I think it's *our* duty to support their decision, no matter how we may feel about the animals it affects." He widened his smile, as though he'd said something quite cheery. "Jane?"

"Oh!" She was caught off guard. "I . . . I'm not sure yet how I feel," she stammered. "I need to think about everything Evie said. I . . . crows are really special to me. If there's any way we could avoid having to, you know . . ." *I sound like a half-wit*, she thought, *even to me*.

"Wow," Katrina intoned. "You'd better figure out where you stand, Jane, or it's gonna be a tough sell for you in the mobile unit." She popped another cookie into her mouth.

"What about you, Avis?" Frank had somehow made himself chair of the impromptu meeting. "You've been here a long time, seen the world come and go." He chuckled at his own way with words.

"I've dedicated the last sixteen years of my life to rescuing animals," Avis responded evenly, "but I'm no good to any of them dead. This West Nile Virus affects the old and the weak first of all, and much as I hate to admit it most of the time, I'm old. And so are a lot of the other long-time volunteers around here." She stuffed the last of her things into her backpack and headed for the door. "One hundred of us care for over three thousand animals every year, year after year. If it came down to numbers alone—and I'm not saying it does, mind you—

it only makes sense to put your volunteers first. As Evie said, do the math!" She stepped outside and slammed the door behind her.

Jane listened to it all, her mind in turmoil. This wasn't extermination. The UWRC wasn't proposing to go out looking for crows to put down. This was humane euthanasia, a compassionate response on the part of any professional rehabilitator to an animal suspected of suffering an irreparable injury or incurable disease. But what about crows that looked healthy? The nestlings and fledges people brought in because they didn't realize the parents were hiding nearby? What about crows hit by cars, or who had hit windows and suffered central nervous system damage? CNS presented just like West Nile, but the recovery rate was much higher. The new policy wouldn't make a distinction between any of them. They'd all be euthanized.

West Nile Virus was on its way—there was no stopping it—and it would arrive in the shape of a crow. What did it mean, Jane asked herself, that the bird whose medicine it was to bring messages from the spirit world to the human realm was approaching with a message about illness? Illness that crossed the boundaries between animals and humans? And what did it mean, she wondered grimly, that they were going to kill the messenger?

Jane found Evie in the exam room writing notes about a cedar waxwing she'd just admitted.

`Hit window — CNS, disoriented, unable to stand or fly. Give fluids, provide standard diet, treat with initial dose of antibiotics to prevent infection, steroids to reduce swelling around brain. Monitor weight, mobility daily.`

She cleared her throat. "Evie..." Evie nodded without looking up from the case sheet. "It's not possible ... you aren't ... the UWRC's decision to euthanize crows doesn't have anything to do with the dead crows that were left outside the door last week. Does it?"

Slowly, Evie lowered her pen to the page and raised blazing eyes to Jane's. "Not one bit." She spoke quietly, but fiercely. "It makes me sick to think that whoever did that might believe we gave in to his threats. What I said in the lunchroom, that was the whole truth. This is about protecting our people and the greatest number of animals possible. End of story." Evie looked down again, sighing. "Sorry if I'm letting my emotions get the upper hand right now, Jane. None of it's directed at you. I hope you know that. Listen, the reason I asked you to see me ... can you do a release this afternoon?"

Whatever Jane had expected to hear, it wasn't that. "Yeah!" She grinned. "I'd love to!" The release was the very last stage of the rehabilitation process. An animal spent days, or sometimes weeks or months, in care at the UWRC, recovering from its injuries or illness and relearning all the skills necessary to survive in the wild: how to forage, hunt, navigate, and fly. For that animal, release was an end to captivity and a return to freedom. For rehabilitators and volunteers, it was the reason for absolutely everything they did, and their greatest reward. "Who gets to go home today?" she asked, excited.

"The crows," Evie answered, her voice ragged with strain. "All of them. Your fledge, too. I'll have them in cardboard kennels, ready to go. Come back after school and get them out of here."

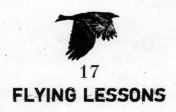

17
FLYING LESSONS

Jane parked in the lower lot at Cedar's Ridge High and cut the engine. It was 4:30 and the lot was almost empty. Cars whizzed by on the road that ran past the school and led up to the ridge, and she found herself praying once more that her little fledge was as ready for flight as Evie believed. It was certainly no match for any predator on the ground. Her six passengers in the back seat were uncharacteristically quiet as she reached in for the fledge's kennel. Taking one last peek at her five remaining charges, she closed the car door and headed across the street.

She set the kennel down on the grass embankment next to the sidewalk and looked up into the branches of the poplars that rose above her. There they were, black shapes camouflaged by afternoon shadows but unmistakable nonetheless. No way to know whether they were the same crows that had scolded her so vehemently the day she'd rescued their little one from the road. Crows spoke in dialects, she knew, and this fledge's ability to survive, to feed, and to find a mate would depend on its ability to communicate with the birds in these trees. Would they speak the same language? All she could do was release him here as she'd promised, and hope.

After giving the fledge a few minutes to acclimate to the sights and sounds of the outdoors after a week inside, Jane tentatively unhooked the flaps at the top of the kennel and spread them wide. The little bird ducked first, as if startled by the immense azure of open sky above him. Then he hopped from the floor of the kennel to the rim and turned on Jane with a mighty "Caah!"

As if they'd been awaiting their cue all week, the crows in the poplars set up an answering ruckus that threatened to blast the leaves from the trees. Over and over they called, until the air was solid sound. An enterprising contingent floated down from the lower branches, landing on the grass a few feet away and casting wary glances at Jane. Continuing to call to the little one, they took turns hopping and leaping into the air, wings beating furiously as they rose into the trees and drifted back down to the ground, up, down, up, down. *A rehabilitator can only do so much*, Jane thought, watching the lesson in wonder. *Wild animals need their own kind.*

Peering over the edge of the kennel, the fledgling at last braved the foot's distance from the rim of the box to the ground, then took a few tentative hops toward its elders, flapping its wings in discovery of a new and latent power. As if crossing some invisible threshold between fledgling and adult, the little crow cast a last look at Jane, hunched, and flew.

Up to the top branches of the poplar the crow rose, and his family with him, until he was simply one of the group, special because she'd rescued him, helped to heal him, but one small black form among so many small black forms, his voice indistinguishable in the ragged song. Jane watched him go, her heart light for the first time that day. Then she returned to her car and headed to the lakeshore with the remaining crows.

Elfin rippled like molten glass in the afternoon heat. Children splashed in the shallows and spun on the merry-go-round at the east end where she'd parked, and picnickers were already laying blankets and firing up hibachis for dinner. Donning sunglasses and a cap, Jane pulled the last two kennels from the backseat and walked the shoreline to a secluded spot at the base of a tall old spruce. Minutes later, she thrilled as five small crows rose together, forgoing the safety of the tree for the moment and choosing instead the freedom of empty sky over the lake. They danced—that was the best word for it, Jane thought as they chased one another, rode the slight breeze, climbed high with no destination and swooped low, just above the surface of the water, feeling the sun on their feathers and the air currents lifting their wings for the first time in their young lives.

Grinning, she stooped to retrieve the empty kennels. When she glanced up again, there were six black shapes against the sky instead of five. She caught her breath and dropped the kennels, her hands flying to her mouth. It was the red-tail.

Soundlessly, upon some invisible signal, the crows had gathered themselves into a tight flock and were making for the sheltering branches of the spruce. They were fast, but the hawk was the more experienced aviator by far. He gained on them with every stroke, until he was twice as close to the crows as they were to the tree.

And then one crow turned and dove for the lake. Jane gasped. *What are you doing?* she wanted to cry out. *You'll never make it!* It never had a chance. But it had known that, it seemed, had chosen to leave the formation to give the rest of them a chance. After a brief chase, the hawk took it in midair, without a sound, and the two plummeted together, disappearing in the field beyond the rushes on the west shore.

And then there were four.

18
UHI

THE FOLLOWING THURSDAY, Jane arrived at the Center just before 8:00 a.m. to find Evie in the middle of the care room with her arms submerged in a tub of steaming water. "More StickiStep victims," she said grimly, nodding her head toward a row of seven cages, each labeled "Rock Pigeon—Oiled" or "Starling—Oiled." She filled two more tubs with water, the little portable generator chugging furiously to keep up with the demand for heat. "Yesterday, we treated six pigeons for poisoning and four the day before. I don't know what's gotten into the people of Cedar's Ridge!"

She shook her head as Jane helped her shift the tubs along the table to make room for towels, gloves, tooth brushes, and dish detergent—all the paraphernalia required to give a bird an oil-spill bath. "It's starting to feel like some kind of conspiracy. First the crows, and then the poisonings, and now this rash of poor, gummed-up pigeons and starlings. I know it's just a coincidence, all of it happening at once like this, but I tell you, it's enough to make a person paranoid." She dipped a thermometer into each of the baths to check the temperature of the water. Satisfied, she pulled on a pair of gloves and reached for the first cage. Dressed head to toe in bright yellow nylon, Jane thought she bore a striking resemblance to Big Bird. She stifled a giggle just in time as Evie pointed to a windbreaker hanging next to the laundry room and said, "Jane, if you think you can stand the heat, suit up. I could really use the help. Daniel's working in the admin office, Beth's on baby birds, Frank and Avis have the outsides covered. Katrina'll have to . . . well, speak of the devil."

"That's a good look on you, Evie," Katrina smiled and batted her lashes as she stepped into the care room. "Seriously, what can I do for you?"

"All of the insides, including fledges, by yourself," Evie said flatly, not responding to the teasing. "As if we're not busy enough already with summer practically here, and on top of eleven patients who need meds this morning, I've got these seven oil-spill baths to do and I'm going to need Jane to assist. Think you can handle it?" Without waiting for an answer, she lifted the first pigeon from his cage and lowered him into the tub.

Jane and Evie worked side by side throughout the morning, and Katrina moved around the perimeter of the room, methodically wrapping birds, cleaning cages, and replacing diets with fresh food. Some small part of Jane's brain registered the opening and closing of cage doors—like a cuckoo clock, she thought, the in and out of birds the only measure of time passing.

Each oiled bird had to be soaped and scrubbed thoroughly, hands working across back, under wings and belly, down the length of tail feathers, and toothbrush finding the tiny spaces along neck, between eyes, across crown, until the water ran clean of oil. Then into the rinse tub, wings extended, right-side-up then upside-down, hose blasting to clear the feathers of soap. Should they miss a patch of oil or soap even the size of a pea, the bird would not be able to recover its insulation and would have to undergo the procedure again—if it survived the first time.

For a time—she didn't know how long—Jane fell into a rhythm alongside Evie, washing, rinsing, setting pigeons under heat to dry, emptying tubs and refilling them in time for the next bird, wiping her face free of sweat. Whenever Katrina had an animal out that required medication, she bundled it up, tapped Evie on the shoulder, and they retreated to the exam room for the few minutes it took to examine, weigh, and treat the patient. In the meantime, Jane continued soaping, massaging, scrubbing, rinsing.

Avis glanced in at some point and left with Frank and Beth, not even bothering to mention break time to Jane and Katrina. Some time later, she returned and stood by the wash table, smelling faintly of coffee and waving two leftover peanut butter cookies under Jane's nose. Jane suddenly realized she was ravenous.

"Well, I should think so!" Avis said curtly. "It's pret'near noon!"

Jane glanced up at the clock—sure enough, it was ten minutes to 12:00—and the whole room flooded back into focus: Katrina, face flushed, hair limp with sweat, making goo-goo faces to an aviary full of reluctant eaters; Evie, drenched head to toe in rinse water; and the one last pigeon cage on the counter.

Jane heard the crunch of gravel as a car pulled into the lot outside. A moment later the front door swung open and closed. Up to her elbows in oily bathwater, her back to reception, she waited to hear Anthony greet the new arrival, but the greeting never came.

"Helloooo!" a woman's high-pitched voice floated down the hallway. "Anyone here?"

Beth was ensconced in ISO1, the door shut tight. Avis and Frank were outside, mucking out the gulls' enclosure, Katrina had ten more minutes on her fledge round, and Evie had just lowered the last pigeon into the tub. "Jane," Evie nodded at her as she squirted another dollop of detergent into the bathwater, "would you mind? If it's anything urgent, just holler and I'll put this guy on standby."

Jane peeled off the fetid windbreaker and tossed it on the laundry pile on her way up the hallway. At reception, she found herself towering over a plump orange mop, permed and hennaed hair styled by wind, apple cheeks fiery with the heat of the day, arms and legs sunned to the color of lobster shells, the entirety garbed in terra cotta polyester shorts and matching tank top. Round blue pools gazed up at her through burgundy-framed glasses as the woman held out a cardboard box: This End Up.

"Babes!" the woman exclaimed in that high, scratchy voice, tears threatening to spill. "I was mowing the lawn, ruddy lazy husband of mine, when I spotted them, poor wee things all alone in the nest, no mother in sight! Orphans!" *UHI, more likely*, Jane thought regretfully, but she kept silent, understanding the woman had done what she thought was best. "I brought them here as soon as I could! Can you save them, then?"

Gently, Jane set the box down on the desk, lifted the lid, and peeked inside. Five impossibly tiny, wizened, gray, featherless, huge-eyed faces gazed back at her. For just a moment, there was silence. And then . . . "*Food! Food! Food! Feed me! Food!*" Jane had no trouble translating, and she grinned down like a fool at the helpless, vulnerable, imperious little creatures. Replacing the lid for the moment, she took up the admissions ledger and admitted them: *June 8 / patients 1168-A, B, C, D, and E / age: juvenile (nestling) / sex: indeterminate / species: _____*. She'd leave that last space for Evie or Daniel to fill in. She guessed they might be starlings or jays.

Jane looked up to find the woman peering anxiously over the reception desk, forehead creased and hands wringing. At once, she heard Anthony's voice in her head, reassuring visitors and callers alike in that warm, funny way of his. It was one of his greatest gifts. Well, she was no Anthony, but she could give it a try.

"They're very, uh, robust-looking," she began, feeling awkward in the role of expert. "I'll put them on heat and we'll add them to the nestling rounds—er, start hand-feeding them in the next fifteen minutes or so." The woman stopped wringing her hands, but her face was still furrowed with worry. "We'll give them every chance, Mrs. . . . uh . . ." she raised her eyebrows, trying out a smile. The woman smiled tentatively back.

"McWhinney. Della McWhinney."

"Tell you what, Mrs. McWhinney," Jane continued, beginning to enjoy the feeling it gave her to see this woman gazing up at her—*Jane Ray, baby bird savior*— "I'll write down their case number for you, 1168, and if you call us, say, next Tuesday or Wednesday, we'll be able to tell you how they're doing."

At this, Della McWhinney beamed, her cheeks going redder than ever. "Oh, ideal! I will do just that! Thank you so much, young lady. You people should be very proud of what you do here!" With that, she pulled a twenty dollar bill from her purse and dropped it in the donation box. Jane gaped, and remembered just in time to thank her as she bustled out through the front door.

Back in the care room, she found a rather limp-looking Evie placing the last pigeon into the drying pen. "Nestlings," she reported. "Five, maybe starlings or jays? I put them on heat, but they seem pretty stable. UHI, probably. Beth should be able to start them on rounds right away."

"Good job, Jane, thanks," Evie answered, giving her a weary smile. "I'll have a look at them as soon as I'm done here." She glanced at the clock: "Hey, it's after noon! You've got school. I'll finish up. You go ahead."

Jane leapt across the wide ditch at the side of the access road and found the narrow dirt path she was looking for, a shortcut that bypassed the smelly, smoggy highway and led through the woods to the school. At its zenith now, the sun had spent its morning warming the trees and the tall grasses, salmonberry bushes, undergrowth, the dirt itself, so that the woods smelled salt-brown-sweet-green with top notes of tang-yellow and berry-pink, as though faeries were cooking their luncheon meal over a thousand small fires. Jane ambled leisurely along the path, feeling a pleasant heaviness in her limbs from the hard work of the morning, and a rumbling in her stomach as she anticipated her own lunch. A picnic on the hill behind the school, maybe, with Amy and Flory and the boys. She'd earned a picnic today, definitely. On a proper blanket. With ice cream from the cafeteria. Pleasant messages about food careened from olfactory to pituitary to stomach to legs, and before she knew it, she was running.

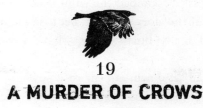

19

A MURDER OF CROWS

JANE GRIPPED THE NEWSPAPER between clenched hands until she thought the bones in her fingers would break. Her eyes swam with tears, her lungs had ceased to breathe, and if her heart had chosen that moment to stop, too, she would not have cared.

It was Wednesday afternoon and when school let out, she, Amy, and Flory had made their way to the Shack to cool off and get a start on a history project that was due at the end of the week. Amy ducked into the underground passage to do a lemonade run, Jane hit the Internet to conduct some preliminary research, and Flory sat at the old wooden table taking dictation and making detailed notes in a fresh black file folder.

Minutes later, Amy had reappeared in the trap door in the floor, red-faced and huffing, bearing a tray of cold drinks and cookies, which she placed on the table. As Jane rose to join the others, Amy pulled a copy of the day's newspaper from under her arm. "Check this out, Jane," she said, passing the paper to her friend with one hand as she divvied up snacks with the other. "Front page, no less! It's too bad the wildlife center didn't get their side of the story out first, because an article like this could really hurt . . . Hey, what's wrong? Jane? Janey?"

Amy had sat down, but she rose now and went immediately to her friend's side. Catching a significant look from Amy, Flory did the same. Something was terribly wrong, something beyond what the article's words seemed to indicate. That was clear from Jane's rigid posture, her stricken face. Glancing anxiously at one another, they waited in silence for their friend to read the story from beginning to end.

CEDAR'S RIDGE CITY HERALD
Animal Sanctuary Destroys Crows Due to West Nile Menace
Wednesday, June 14

LOWER MAINLAND—It was, in the most brutal sense of the word, a murder of crows.

For several days, North Vancouver residents Della and Norm McWhinney watched a nest of crow hatchlings in their backyard. The five chicks were active from dawn til dusk, waking the McWhinneys each morning with calls for food and commandeering the activities of two doting parents.

"The parents were never far away," Della McWhinney said Tuesday. "They brought those little ones bugs and all the whole day long."

But when the two adult crows disappeared for over three hours last week, the McWhinneys assumed the worst. "We took matters into our own hands," said Norm McWhinney. "We'd been to the Urban Wildlife Rescue Center before and had every confidence they'd know what to do."

Mrs. McWhinney delivered the five chicks to the UWRC and was instructed to phone the Center in a few days to check on the birds' condition. When she did, she was told they had been euthanized immediately after admission as a matter of policy. "I couldn't believe my ears," she said, in tears.

Because the threat of West Nile Virus looms over BC, the UWRC has implemented a new policy whereby all crows brought to the shelter are immediately destroyed and their bodies delivered to officials at the Province's animal health center for examination.

West Nile affects hundreds of bird species, but corvids are the indicator species, meaning the virus will appear in them first. They also have an extremely low survival rate and are potential carriers that could transmit the virus to other animals in the shelter.

UWRC spokesperson Evelyn Jordan said today, "In order to protect other patients in our care, as well as our staff and volunteers, we made the decision to humanely euthanize any crows that are brought to us between now and the end of September."

"I was devastated," Della McWhinney said after learning her "rescued" crows had been destroyed. "There wasn't a thing wrong with them! If I'd known what those people were going to do, I would never have left those little birds there to die."

Not starlings. Not jays. Crows. They'd been crows. *My fault.*

Why hadn't she asked someone? Anyone? Called for Evie? Checked a reference book for photos of hatchlings? Asked the woman if *she* knew what they were. Asked her if she was absolutely sure the parents weren't coming back. Anything. *Anything.* But Jane had done none of those things. Her mind raced through the list of things she hadn't done, as though by thinking them fast enough she might somehow turn back the clock and relive those three minutes at the reception counter with Della McWhinney.

My fault.

"Murder," the reporter had called it. What a terrible twist, that the media should have chosen to portray the Center's decision this way, while someone in the community had gotten away with the deliberate and brutal killing of crows. The Center operated on the kindness and goodwill of the community. An article like this could cripple it if people couldn't see past the sensationalism to the real reasons behind the UWRC's policy.

My fault. My fault.

The music-box melody of an ice-cream truck floated in from the road behind the house, ridiculously incongruous in light of what lay in her hands. Jane was trembling, she realized, and her legs were about to give way. She hadn't drawn a breath since Amy had handed her the newspaper. She looked up at Amy and Flory then, tears spilling from her eyes, her mouth open in a soundless cry. *My fault!* she wanted to cry out. *This is my fault!*

And then she heard it, over the hum of the computer, the beating of her own heart, the ice-cream song. It was the caahing of crow nestlings in a tree somewhere nearby, demanding to be fed. And if she'd thought she could do no worse than betray Evie and the Center with her careless mistake, now she knew she was wrong.

And she was lifting the lid again—This End Up— and peeking in. And the five were looking up at her, eyes and mouths wide, healthy, vulnerable, *alive.*

And then there were none.

Her knees buckled and she fell into the chair. Amy and Flory rushed to place their hands on her back and press their bodies close to her, as though to hold her together. "It was me," she managed to force the words out in a small, strangled voice, hoping they would understand what she meant. Then she lay her head down on the wooden table and sobbed.

20
ANIMAL RIGHTS...AND WRONGS

A MILE FROM THE WILDLIFE CENTER, Jane pulled
over and shut off her car, unable to go any further.
Thursday morning had dawned clear and searingly
hot, and as she forced herself through the motions of
getting ready for her shift at the UWRC, it occurred
to her more than once that real weather, unlike movie
weather, often did a poor job of reflecting one's mood.
Twice she'd reached for the phone, with the intention
of calling in sick. And twice she'd changed her mind,
knowing that "sick at heart" didn't count, that newspaper articles didn't mean anything to the animals
waiting to be fed, and that if she had to face Evie's disappointment or her anger, she'd be wise not to put it off
another whole week.

But when she rounded the first curve on the long
access road that wound through the woods and down
to the shore of Aerie Lake, she realized that the incident
with Della McWhinney and its aftermath was no longer
hers to face alone. The skewed story in yesterday's newspaper had been picked up by radio and television outlets

across the city, and its echoes had reached thousands—many of them animal lovers—who heard only the decision to euthanize crows and not the reasons behind it. The story had galvanized people into action in a way that much bigger stories often failed to do. Between Wednesday dusk and Thursday dawn, the access road had filled to choking with cars, tents, and sleeping bags, placards and handmade signs, news cameras, and marching bodies all shouting, vying for the next sound-bite, the next clip, the last word.

ANIMAL KILLERS! many of the signs read.

UWRC DUPES PUBLIC! read several others.

CROW KILLERS!

I WANT MY MONEY BACK!

KILL THEIR FUNDING!

PULL THE PLUG!

UWRC KILLS PATIENTS!

ANIMAL RESCUE? NOT HERE!

EUTHANIZE THE UWRC!

It was a mob scene.

Jane sat perfectly still inside her car, windows rolled up, hands gripping the steering wheel, eyes following a large woman in a sun suit and flip flops who was screaming obscenities at one of the television crew as she set a wooden birdhouse on fire. The crowd roared as the flames caught, and Jane watched little fires start all down the length of the road as people set about to imitate the woman's dramatic gesture. *It would take one errant spark,* she thought, *to set the whole woods aflame.* For a month now, it had been dry, and hot. *Just one spark.*

She was shaking now, and rivers of acrid sweat slid down her face, ran the length of her neck, beaded under her arms and slithered down her torso. *Fear,* some small, rational part of her mind said. *This is what I smell like when I'm afraid.*

She leaned forward and reached for the ignition key, her brain on auto-pilot and her body concerned with one thing only: getting away. But the small movement brought another parked car into view that had been partially hidden by the bend in the road. A car she knew. Evie's car. Empty. Which meant that Evie had walked from here to the Center. Had walked through this crowd to get to the animals. They needed food, fresh water, medication, today just like any other day. The Center was open three hundred and sixty-five days a year, and it was either Evie or Daniel who unlocked the door each morning.

Jane pulled her keys from the ignition and stuffed them into the pocket of her backpack. Her hand brushed a familiar object, and she drew it out: her UWRC nametag. Yes. If she was going to do this, she might as well do it right. Pinning the small plastic tag to her shirt, she stepped out of her car, swung her backpack over her shoulders and started to walk.

It was the longest mile of her life.

The wave of sound started somewhere near the parked cars and traveled the length of the road ahead of her with frightening speed. Jane understood that somehow, the two or three thousand protestors picketing the road were communicating with one another using these undercurrents of sound, and that it was now known from here to the Center that another volunteer was on her way up the road. As she stepped into the throng, she felt the heat of the day trebled by the heat of bodies and the heat of their anger. Her clothing was soaked with sweat, and she had three thousand steps to go. *So, okay, go. One at a time. Go. Just keep going.*

Bodies pressed close, men and women and even some children, waving their arms and their signs, shouting insults and taunts. She kept her eyes facing ahead and slightly down, on the road, on her path, on her next destination, this bulrush and then that salmonberry bush and then that alder tree. But she couldn't shut her ears. "Are you proud of yourself, you crow-killer?" "What part of 'rescue' do you not understand?" "You should be ashamed, euthanizing innocent, healthy animals!" "Is this what you spend our donations on?" "We're going to sue you!" "We'll bleed you dry!" "How do you get to decide who dies?" "Those who kill the innocent deserve to die themselves!"

Shocks pulsed through her body as she heard the words. Her breathing came shallow and fast, her face was hot with fear and exertion, and her heart hammered so that she thought it must show to all these people who wanted to make her afraid. *Do. Not. Cry.* She said a word to herself with each step, over and over again. *Keep. Going. Do. Not. Cry.*

In the periphery of her vision, she saw Police Chief Emery pull apart two men by the far ditch who had graduated from shouts to blows. *Police. So that's why they don't kill me,* she thought. *Because they* want *to.*

Police or no police, the mob certainly wanted to hurt her. Glancing up to get her bearings, she estimated she had about a hundred and fifty yards to go, when the stone hit her back. Without a thought, she whirled and hunched like a cornered animal. There was nowhere to run, so she would fight. Her eyes widened in surprise when she spotted the small boy winding up to throw a second rock. A man in his thirties, presumably the boy's father, stood close by, making no effort to restrain the child. He narrowed his eyes, taking in Jane's sweaty, disheveled appearance, her obvious fear. "You goody-goody types," he shouted at her, "take the public's money and what do you do with it? What are you teaching our children about animals? About *compassion?*" Not waiting to hear any more, or to find out where the second rock would land, she spun on her heel and ran.

Rounding the last curve in the road and seeing the Center looking peaceful as always, surrounded by gardens and nesting birds and lakeshore, she almost cried out in relief. But she choked off the sound and skidded to a stop as she realized her beloved little Center had been ravaged during the night.

Ugly scrawls of black spray paint scarred the outside of the Center, and several of the animal outbuildings as well. The "artist" had been more succinct than the sign-makers, sticking to a repertoire of MURDER and CROW KILLERS on every building. All of the windows in the Center had been smashed, and hastily covered from the inside, Jane saw, with sheets of scrap plastic and paper. One final sign hung from the old apple tree in the garden, the words underscored with an arrow pointing to the front door: THIS WAY TO DIE. She didn't know how long she stood there, staring, but suddenly another fast-approaching tsunami of sound from the crowd on the road reached her ears, and with the time for hesitation past, she strode to the door and stepped inside.

Whatever greeting she'd anticipated from Evie this morning, she certainly never expected a homecoming. "Jane! Thank goodness you're safe!" Evie cried from behind the reception desk. And she rushed to Jane and wrapped her arms around her and held her as though she might never let go.

"I'm so sorry," Jane choked out through tears, crying now against Evie's shoulder. "I'm so sorry, Evie."

"Hush." Evie patted her back gently, but the word was a command. "This is not your fault." She gripped

Jane by the shoulders and took a step back, looking directly into her eyes. Jane noticed she was pale and drawn, her mouth held tight in a thin white line. "This is poor timing and communication on our part and irresponsible reporting on the part of the media. If this is anybody's fault, it's mine. I should never have let you do that intake on your own."

"Right, Evie, it's your fault," Daniel broke in, trying for a smile. For the first time, Jane noticed that virtually the whole Thursday morning crew was gathered around the computer and phones at reception like soldiers under siege gathering at their command station. The usual smells of animal feces, food, and antiseptic were overlayed with the scent of fear—human fear. "And Anthony blames himself for being away from his desk, and Beth blames herself for not hearing the door last week . . . You know, I think we've got enough people in the enemy camp to last us a lifetime," he said, nodding in the direction of the road. "Let's drop the fault-finding and the blaming and just deal with what's on our plates, okay? We're going to have to stick together to get through this." With that, he stepped into the exam room and began drawing up meds for the morning's patients. Jane was reminded once more of the reason they were all here: the animals.

The phone rang as Katrina and Beth turned to follow his lead and get started on their rounds. Anthony made a comical face at the telephone, but not before Jane noticed he'd jumped at the sound. She'd seen people on the road with cell phones in their hands. Were they tying up the animal help line to call in with their jeers and threats?

Anthony relaxed visibly when he heard the voice on the other end. "Of course, baby! No way, uh-uh! You go home and you tell them Anthony said so! Really, hon, we've got enough people here. You go, and we'll see you next week, okay? Okay, bye." He sighed as he replaced the receiver, and then looked up at Evie. "Avis. Must have found a pay phone somewhere. Can you imagine? Poor thing actually contemplated walking that gauntlet. At her age! Bloody heathens!" he finished with a wave of his hand in the direction of the road. "Terrifying little old ladies!"

"Not to mention young ones," Jane muttered, gingerly rubbing the spot on her back where the stone had hit her. "Hey Anthony, where's Frank?" He was the only other member of the regular crew she hadn't seen.

Evie scowled. "Not here." She shared a cryptic look with Daniel. "I don't think he'll be in."

"Maybe when things die down . . . ?" Anthony ventured.

"Ever." Evie drummed her fingers hard on the reception counter, then slammed her hand down. "Dammit! I did the reference checks, called his previous employers, everything! I mean, I knew he was a passionate animal rights guy, but I never would have . . ." She let the sentence trail off as she covered her face with her hands.

"I . . . I don't understand," Jane stammered, not sure if this conversation was meant for her ears or not. She would be summer staff by the end of the month, but still . . . She looked up to find Daniel staring thoughtfully at her.

"Turns out Frank's a pretty hard-core animal rights guy," Daniel began. Jane shook her head at him, frowning. So? She'd call herself an animal rights person, too. With a quick glance at Evie, Daniel pressed on. "Someone the authorities have labeled an eco-terrorist. That graffiti out there isn't his first act of vandalism, apparently. He's left quite a collection of exploded cars and burned-down buildings in his wake. We got off easy, I understand."

Jane gasped, trying to force the things Daniel was saying to make sense. She failed. "Why?" she pleaded, looking from Daniel to Evie. "Why would he do that to us? I thought he agreed with your . . . I don't understand . . . how on earth can vandalism and violence help animals?"

"You tell me," Daniel answered grimly. "Or better yet, go tell our friends on the road, the 'animal lovers' who'd apparently rather see us dead than protecting our patients and our people." He shook his head, weary with arguing a case he couldn't win, and turned his attention back to the meds board.

"I nearly forgot . . . we did get one piece of good news this morning!" Evie's falsely cheerful voice rang hollow in the tension of the reception area, but Jane forced herself to play along. She had four hours of this siege to get through, but the staff had a full day ahead of them, and then tomorrow, and then the next day. They would need to use every means at hand to keep their spirits up in the face of this public onslaught.

"What's that, Evie?" Jane asked, trying to match her light tone. "You guys win the lottery pool?"

"Kind of!" was Evie's surprising answer. "We'd been waiting for a decision from City Council on a grant we applied for. Couple of months ago, now. We figured it was a lost cause. But last week, Councilor Harbinsale re-tabled the proposal and they voted, and we're getting the money!"

"And none too soon, girlfriend," Anthony shot back over his shoulder as he scanned the day's emails. "That puts us at one for six, hmm?"

Evie crumpled, her bravado suddenly gone and her small victory with it. "Right, yeah, one for six. I'm going to get the laundry started."

As Evie retreated slowly down the hallway, Anthony bent forward and dropped his head into his hands. Tentatively, Jane placed a light hand on his shoulder. "What's wrong, Anthony? What just happened?" The communiqués were flying faster than she could keep up, most of them without benefit of words.

"We lost five corporate donors this morning," came the muffled answer. "Major ones. And I just dumped a big bucket of cold water on Evie's one good thing." He swiveled suddenly in his chair to face Jane, looking close to tears. "But not just corporate ones, Jane girl, individuals, too! Wonderful people who've been donating for years, suddenly pulling their money because they think we've gone crazy! And who can blame them? The way they made us look on the news yesterday, I'd do the same!" He swung slowly around to face the computer again. "We run this place on those people's donations," he said, his voice barely more than a whisper. "If something doesn't give, this could shut us down forever."

"So this City grant is a really good thing, then," she ventured, trying to bring the focus back around to something positive. "And Councilor Harbinsale pushing it through, of all people!"

"Yeah, go figure," Anthony said, still cynical. "That man is poison when it comes to animals and the environment. But right now, he's our savior. I never thought I'd see the day, I must say."

Jane made her way to the care room to take a count of the fledglings, then headed into the kitchen to start their diets. No one spoke this morning, she noticed, but instead went about their work in silence, no energy to spare for niceties or social banter, every effort focused on shutting out the noise of the crowd and getting through the morning's tasks. Even the animals were mostly silent, clearly attuned to both the threat that lay outside and the tension the caregivers carried with them inside. Jane missed Avis's bustling presence, her no-nonsense manner, even her crabby complaints and criticisms.

All of the rooms were darker than usual and stiflingly hot, the smashed windows covered over roughly with sheets of plastic and cardboard. It felt safer, being invisible to the people outside, but strange not to see the light, not to be able to look out at the lake as she prepared the food, to watch the birds in their aviaries, just one step away from wild. She was reminded of something she'd read in a history textbook, about air-raid drills during the Second World War: the siren would blare, rousing you from peace and from whatever ordinary thing you'd been doing, and you'd have to run from room to room making sure every window was blacked out, every light was shut off, so that when the enemy came, the bomber pilot would not be able to see your home in the dark. Those who'd been children during the war never forgot the feeling of terror brought on by the air-raid siren, even if the bomb never came, even if all they ever experienced was a drill.

Today is not a drill, Jane thought.

"This has to be the worst week of my life," Katrina muttered as she pushed her way into the kitchen and slammed the door behind her. She was looking after all the outside pens by herself today, just as Jane was managing the care room by herself. "Mike can't come get me til his spare this afternoon, which means I miss gym class. But there is no way I'm walking through that nut farm again alone." Jane closed her eyes, remembering what it was like to have someone just a phone call away, ready to face the dragons by her side. "And now he's cancelled all our weekend plans to go to some engineering info session at the university. I mean, it's great that he's keen and all, but we had *three* parties to go to! And I am *so* not going alone." Her heart sinking, Jane turned from the counter to ask her more, but she was gone.

Reaching up to the dry goods shelf for the wild birdseed, her hand landed in empty space. Peanuts, sunflower seeds, wheat and corn mix . . . no wild birdseed. Maybe Daniel had it in the exam room. She paused in the laundry room to switch loads and empty the dryers. Despite the heat, they would put nothing to dry on the outside lines today. She would have walked right by Anthony at reception and into the exam room, except that her mind somehow registered what he was doing: he was on the UWRC website, working in html, erasing Evie Jordan's name. She stood stock still and silent behind him as he went on to erase Daniel's name and then his own.

Suddenly he became aware of her presence, and spun around with a start. "Oh, Jane girl," he said miserably. "Nobody was supposed to see."

Her mind reeled. Was this more vandalism? Could it be? Was Anthony in on it, too? "Now, before you jump to any dastardly conclusions," he said, guessing her thoughts, "let me just say I am acting on official orders." He nodded pertly, as though he'd explained everything.

"But why?" she breathed, that feeling of overwhelming confusion threatening to overtake her once again.

Anthony stared at her hard, his lips pursed. "You can't tell, Jane. I wasn't supposed to let anybody know. We didn't want the volunteers to get scared."

"Oh, Anthony, if you knew how scared I am already that would be almost funny!" Jane replied, her voice rising with panic.

"Easy, girl," he said in a soothing voice, holding his hands out in front of him. "It's just . . . it's just that there's been a . . ." He stopped to clear his throat and take a deep breath. "Death threat. There. I said it. A death threat. Against Evie. This morning. Some lunatic, for sure. The police are on it. Nothing to worry about, probably, they said. But they thought maybe the website . . . it has everybody's name on it, see. So I'm taking them off. The names." He let out his breath in a quiet hiss. "Might not stop the death threats, but at least from now on, they won't start 'Dear Evie Jordan.'"

The phone rang, startling them both. "Urban Wildlife Rescue, how may I . . . oh, hi! Oh, lady, I'm glad it's you."

Numb, Jane walked slowly back down the hallway before remembering she'd been on her way to the exam room. She turned and retraced her steps, arriving at the exam room door with no recollection of why she'd come in the first place. Behind her, she heard Anthony call Evie to the phone. In front of her, Daniel stood at the exam table, an injured sparrow in his hands. She looked up at Daniel, her eyes full of tears. One spilled over the lid and splashed onto her hand. "I don't know why I'm here!" she said, her voice little more than a whisper. "I forget why I'm here!"

Daniel held her gaze, the expression on his face mirroring her feelings exactly, and took a slow, deep breath. She found herself doing the same. "For the animals," he answered softly.

Jane was rinsing the last of the dirty dishes when Evie came into the kitchen. "Looking for me?" Jane asked, venturing a smile. The morning's routines had calmed and grounded her, and in spite of everything, she was glad she'd come today.

"As a matter of fact, yes," Evie said, trying unsuccessfully to return the smile. "We had a phone call . . ."

Jane felt her stomach plummet and her heart start to race. Was there no end? *Today is not a drill.*

"Another sponsor, uh, withdrew support because of the new policy." Evie looked at the ceiling, took a deep breath, and then looked directly at Jane. "We lost the car. We lost the new staff positions. There won't be a transport team this summer. I'm sorry."

She rushed on before Jane could interject. "You'll still have a job! That is, if we still look like an attractive employer to you." Her smile took the form of an awkward scowl. "I can offer you Frank's hours in animal care. Just . . . just no transport team. I'm so sorry, Jane."

Without thinking, Jane rushed forward and wrapped her arms around a surprised Evie. After a moment, Evie hugged her back, hard. "Sign me up," was all she said.

Evie laughed, a choked sound but the first real sign of light in her all morning. "Well, all right then!" Together, they walked up the hallway to reception.

As she packed up her knapsack in preparation to leave, Jane suddenly realized she was the only person who would have to make the trip out alone. Mike was coming later for Katrina, and the rest of the crew would walk back to their cars together. Daniel must have arrived at the same thought at the same moment. He stepped out of the exam room, grabbing his T-shirt and jeans on the way. "Give me two minutes to get out of these scrubs, Jane, and I'll go with you."

She shook her head before she had time to think about it. "Either *I* go alone now, or *you* come back alone later. How is one better than the other?" she asked rhetorically, her voice firm. "Besides, it's a mile, and as you well know, I can do a mile in eight minutes . . . if I run!" Inside, she was quaking, but on the outside she managed a sort of lopsided grin. Grudgingly, Daniel grinned back.

"Well, at the risk of sounding like your mother, call us when you get to school, will you?" he said.

Jane nodded. She reached down to unpin her nametag, then changed her mind. With a little wave of her hand to Evie, Daniel, and Anthony, she slung her pack over her shoulders and stepped outside. They spotted her instantly—a pack of hungry wolves who'd waited too long in the midday heat for sight of their prey. She felt the rumblings start, the beginning of that tidal wave of sound. *If I run fast enough,* she wondered, her preoccupation with the challenge momentarily drowning out the clamor of fear, *could I outrun the wave?*

She trained her eyes on the sight of the sun streaming through the trees, and her ears on the songs of the birds that lived and mated and nested in their branches, and she ran so fast the tears dried on her cheeks before they could fall.

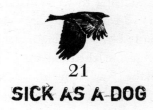

21
SICK AS A DOG

BEFORE SHE OPENED HER EYES, Jane wondered what on earth her mother had done with her bones. She had a vague recollection of her mom's hand on her forehead, her shoulders, her ankles. That must have been when she'd done it—taken them out and baked them dry. But then she'd put them back wrong: leg bones in her arms, stretching the skin to the tearing point; arm bones in her legs, much, much too small. Everything the wrong size in the wrong place, everything hurting, so that she couldn't move her own body, even shift her weight, without fear of breaking apart entirely. It was too late for her head, that much she knew for sure. It was being crushed to pulp by the beauty-parlor-style hairdryer they'd attached to it, the setting on High and much too tight. She could feel her scalp molding itself to the bones of her skull as it melted.

Everything was red and shades of red—scarlet, russet, fire, and blood. *If I could just work these eyeballs for a minute,* she thought, *I could see the other colors. I know there are other colors.* One lid lifted, then the other, the two refusing to work in tandem. She felt herself floating in a white skiff, pale, watery surroundings undulating in a rhythm that matched the throbbing pulse of her mismatched bones. A gigantic Raggedy Anne doll sat at the prow, facing into the boat instead of toward shore. *Stop staring at me,* Jane thought crossly, unable to make herself heard over the roar of the hair dryer. The ocean breeze caught Raggedy Anne's monstrous mane of wooly orange curls and the doll began to pitch forward, as though she was about to topple from her perch and land atop Jane's fragile bones. She closed both eyes at once and lay perfectly still, not breathing, waiting for the crushing weight to fall. When at last she opened them again, the doll was gone.

Some time later, she tried again, first one eye, then the other. This time, it was Wednesday Addams from the Addams family who had taken up her position as the backward-facing figurehead. Suddenly, Jane understood—*she* was a cartoon character, too! Not real at all. That was why everything ached and throbbed. They'd probably been drawing and erasing her, stretching her out long and squishing her down flat with special effects, tossing her off cliffs with anvils and filling her full of holes with a long-barreled shotgun. *Cartoon characters must be expected to do their own stunts around here,* she thought. *Well, I'll check my contract. I want to make sure I'm getting paid for it.* With that, she closed her eyes once more, and slept.

Flory marched smartly alongside Ms. Adani, stopping at desks and inside office doors to shake hands and commit faces and names to memory as she was introduced. The formal part of her orientation tour at City Hall was coming to an end, and her soon-to-be supervisor was ushering her down the corridor that led to the offices of the City Councilors, and the Mayor, for the final introductions. Despite this, she was no longer nervous at all. They'd run into Mayor Barney in the lunchroom, assembling the ingredients of a veggie pita wrap and microwaving his lentil soup. He invited her to join him before comprehending that she was in the middle of her orientation and so offered her a raincheck for another day. She'd accepted with delight. His jovial welcome and down-to-earth manner instantly put her at ease. She was going to love working here, she just knew it.

Ms. Adani knocked on several closed doors and got no response. Flory noted the names: Gunnarson, Hatch, Moody, Parmar, Tierza. "Oh, Flory, I'm terribly sorry, it looks as if most of the councilors are out for lunch. We'll just have to pick up where we left off when you arrive next week for your first day of work. Meanwhile, why don't you and I run across the street to the Poivre Bistro!" She smiled warmly, and Flory congratulated herself again on landing the ideal summer job.

Suddenly, one of the closed doors swung open and there, standing in the doorway and filling the frame, was Rand Harbinsale. "Councilor Harbinsale!" Ms. Adani exclaimed. "How fortuitous! We thought you'd all stepped out. Oh, and Councilor Moody, I didn't see you there. What luck!" Flory could see a small female form hovering behind the desk in the shadows of the office. She almost laughed, realizing she could have recognized the woman based exclusively on Jane's description of her. Recovering quickly, she stepped forward and held out her hand to Councilor Harbinsale.

"Flory Morales, Councilors. One of the new summer interns. City parks and environmental operations. I'm very pleased to meet you both!" Dying of curiosity was more like it, but she'd mind her manners—for the time being. She was gratified to see that Councilor Harbinsale didn't recognize her. Of course, on the occasion of their first meeting, she'd been disguised rather effectively as a diving duck.

"Miss Morass!" Rand grasped her hand and held on, smiling down at the petite girl in a rather discomfiting way.

"That's 'Morales,' sir."

"Right, yes. Excellent timing. Madge and I were just discussing a very important document that will be put forward again at the next Council meeting. As you may have heard we have proposed to declare Cedar's Ridge a 'Pest-Free City!'" He beamed. "You're just in time to join the team and help us put the plan into action! Isn't that right, Madge? What say we add Miss Morass here to the team!" He was still pumping Flory's hand.

"'Morales,' sir."

"Oh, Councilor Harbinsale," Ms. Adani began, a look of deep concern shadowing her face. "I thought Council had recommended . . ."

"Now, slow down, Rand," interrupted a prim voice from inside the office. "It's still in the proposal stages. There's no guarantee Council will go for it next time either." Flory detected a note of false modesty in Madge Moody's voice. The woman obviously thought their proposal for a pest-free Cedar's Ridge was a hands-down winner. For her part, Flory thought the two of them must be crazy. A round, curl-covered head poked itself through the doorway, well below the level of Rand Harbinsale's shoulder. Intense, round eyes looked Flory up and down and all the way back up again. Flory, meanwhile, kept a bland smile on her face and willed herself to hold the woman's gaze. "And until they do," Councilor Moody finished, a tiny smile on her own face, "we do *not* require any more *team* members."

"The vote was five to four, Madge—we're almost there! Besides, no need to wait for the whole city to get started," Rand pressed on, still smiling at Flory. "The Country Club I manage is already a pest-free zone, as is my own home estate. Even the local wildlife shelter has gotten in on the act—without any prompting on my part, I might add!—helping to rid this city of an unsightly *and* unhealthy nuisance. And they earned themselves a nice fat grant out of the deal. You see, if we all do our part, Cedar's Ridge will be the most livable city in the Lower Mainland, if not the province! Maybe even the country!"

Flory was appalled by Harbinsale's take on the UWRC's policy with respect to crows, but she kept her expression neutral, and seized the opening. "What sorts of pests are you planning to get rid of, sir?" she inquired, an expression of what she hoped was dumb innocence fixed on her face. "Will you start with homeless people?"

She waited for the coughing to subside before she continued. "Or were you thinking more like bugs and stuff? They *are* pretty creepy, hey! Although, if you kill all the bugs dead, there won't be anybody to pollinate the plants *and* that'll make the birds die off, cuz I mean, what are the birds going to eat? Oh, but maybe you meant *birds!* They *can* be pretty pesky, actually, those darn birds, waking you up at the crack of dawn and pooping all over your car and everything! Or maybe you were meaning rodents? Like rats and mice? Course, then eagles and hawks have nothing to eat so they die off, too. But that could be good because . . . well, actually, maybe that wouldn't be good cuz they keep the rodent populations under control, don't they? So yeah, not so good. Hmmm . . . what about coyotes? Oh, wait, no—same deal with the rodents." Eyes wide and face utterly serious, she gave a low whistle, in full performance mode now. "Wow, sirs! I mean, sir and ma'am. A pest-free city! So, like, what's your strategy?"

Rand Harbinsale gazed down at her. His smile was undiminished but his eyes had turned to steel. "Well, now, aren't you just the little livewire! Here for the whole summer, is she, Ms. Adani? Hmmm, yes. Well, then, Miss *Morales*, perhaps I could take you for lunch some time to . . . discuss that strategy. I'd love to know a little more about your, er, philosophy."

Flory's "creep" radar instantly sent alarm bells clanging through her brain. She'd eat bugs herself before she'd let Rand Harbinsale take her anywhere for lunch. But all she said was, "That would be lovely, sir. The Mayor just invited me to do the same. Perhaps we could all bring sandwiches on the same day." With a nod, she turned in unison with Ms. Adani, but not before she saw the councilor's jaw drop.

They stepped into the elevator and as the doors rolled shut, Ms. Adani stared up at the floor numbers, an irrepressible grin lighting her whole face. "I had a feeling we were going to hit it off when I hired you, Flory Morales," she said without looking down. Now I know why. I do believe I can die a happy woman, having seen that look on Rand Harbinsale's face."

Better than a candy store, was the thought that kept running through Amy's head. *Better than rainbow gumballs and blue freezies, better than two-cent sours, better than toffees or gummies or nickel peppermint patties or miniature licorice jawbreakers.* She inhaled a deep breath of antiseptic and bleach, and exhaled, in nirvana. A real laboratory.

Spotless white surfaces accessorized with gleaming surgical steel. Shelves stocked with an orderly assortment of medicine vials, ointments, pill bottles, homeopathics, and herbals, organized by type of medication and then alphabetically, everything in its place. Scales that measured weight to the tenth of a gram, and microscopes that magnified by a thousand times. Spectrometers, centrifuges, slides, syringes, scalpels, forceps, and surgical scissors. Splints, bandages, and adhesives. Incubators and x-ray equipment. Real lab coats. And in the middle of it all, Amy Airlie MacGillivray. Scientist. Oooohh, that sounded good. Maybe they'd whip her up some business cards.

She was pleased to note that her own lab in the Shack wasn't entirely lame by comparison, but oh . . . this was heaven. She popped her head into the corridor. The coast was clear. Her supervisor had left her alone for a moment to retrieve some official summer-employee paperwork for her to sign. Finally, she could do what she'd been dreaming of ever since her orientation had begun that morning. Leaping into the air, she catapulted silently but energetically through the entire halftime routine of the Cedar's Ridge Senior Secondary Cheerleading Squad. The whole summer. Here. And on top of it all, they were going to *pay* her. Oooh baby, life was sweet.

Jane took another sip of hot water from her mug and then lay weakly back against the pillows. Her fever had broken, finally, which meant she was on the mend, but she had a few more days of daytime television and afternoon naps with the kitties ahead of her before she'd be a hundred percent. Sweet Pea and Minnie gazed at her imperturbably from the foot of the bed, one perched on Amy's lap and the other on Flory's. This was the first time she was aware of having visitors, but according to her mom, her friends had come by every day since she'd fallen sick.

"So your jobs are fabulous?" she asked, grinning. "Tell me everything again. At least I can live vicariously through you two."

"Oh, Jane, that is no contest the worst news ever about your transport job," Amy commiserated. "Flory and I were *so* looking forward to being driven all over town in your sassy little hybrid car!"

"It's okay, Jane, we'll still ride with you. Your sedan is very sexy," Flory said seriously. Jane and Amy broke out into peals of laughter.

"Boy magnet!" Jane wheezed. "I can hardly go anywhere without being propositioned!"

"By who?" Amy wheezed, the tears starting. "Spare parts dealers?"

Catching her breath, Jane said, "You know, it's going to be weird, us doing three different things this summer. I think I'm going to miss you guys!"

"We'll still have weekends at Cultus," Amy said practically, wiping her eyes on her arm. "And besides, it'll give us more to talk about when we meet at the Shack after work."

"Yes, because we so often run out of things to say," Flory added, straightfaced. There was a pause while the other two digested what she'd said, and then they were all laughing again.

"I can't believe I'm missing the end of my grade eleven year!" Jane said finally. "I just hope I'm all better in time to start work at the UWRC." She paused. "You know, I'm worried this is getting to be a Jane Ray thing . . ."

"What do you mean, Jane?" Flory leaned forward, intrigued by her friend's cryptic remark.

"Getting sick, crashing when I'm stressed," Jane replied. "I came close to bowing out of the fight with SeaKing last year, remember? And now, with the wildlife center under attack . . . I mean, I've missed my last two shifts! There couldn't be a worse time for me to be away. They need all the support they can get right now, and here I am in bed. In fact, I'm sure there are people who think I'm making some kind of statement against the Center's policy by staying away." She sighed, frowning into her mug of tepid water. "My heart's there, but my body seems to have had other ideas."

"That is the single dumbest thing I've ever heard," Amy retorted, snorting for emphasis. "You've been half-dead with the flu for over a week, and if . . ."

"*Are* you making a statement, Jane?" Flory interrupted, very quietly.

Jane raised her eyes to meet her friend's, but found no judgment there, only curiosity. "I . . . I don't know, Flor," she answered just as quietly, realizing she was testing the idea out loud for the first time. "My head tells me that of all the possible options, this policy is the best one for the greatest number of animals and people." She paused, setting her mug on the bedside table and rubbing the fingers of one hand with the other. "But my heart asks, 'What about the individual crows? What about those unique lives, their favorite trees, their joy in flying, their mates and their young, their desires and plans?" She shook her head, as though staring at some unfathomable algebra equation. "There should be a solution that works for the individuals *and* for the whole, but I can't think what it could be. And meanwhile, I guess, my body is torn between the two."

Flory nodded, seeming to understand. Amy merely snorted again. "What a load of crap!" she said, catapulting Sweet Pea off her lap as she made her point. "You've been sick as a dog, Jane! Nobody can blame you for taking some time off, or say it's some sort of protest. And speaking of dogs, by the way, if it's any consolation, Buster's been sick, too. Barfing up a storm. And I highly doubt it's because he's feeling emotionally conflicted about the political situation at the UWRC!"

Jane giggled at that, suddenly feeling immensely better. Flory's willingness to hear her out coupled with Amy's refusal to take her too seriously were just the medicine she'd needed. "So I guess you'll have to figure out how to have fun at Cultus without me this weekend," she teased. "I don't think I'm up for the long drive just yet."

"Actually," Amy responded, exchanging glances with Flory, "it's Mike's grad weekend, and my parents will be at Cultus, so I'm sticking around to keep an eye on Buster."

Flory nodded, glancing at Amy again. "Uh-huh, me too, sticking around, I mean. I'm going to type up some notes on my orientation and get a file started on City Hall. I've got some ideas about how to increase apartment-block participation in the city's recycling program."

Jane looked back and forth at her two best friends, eyes narrowed with suspicion. "Exactly what is with the mysterious glances, you two? Hello, yes, I saw! I may be sick, but I'm not brain-dead."

"Nothing!" Flory squeaked lamely.

"She's right, Jane," Amy concurred, "it's nothing, really. Just . . . the Mike thing . . . you know, grad, Katrina . . . We were hoping not to bring it up, because we know you kind of like him, and with . . ."

"*What?*" Jane was suddenly fully alert, and her cheeks burned as though the fever might be threatening to reassert itself. "Like *Mike?* As in, *like* like? Your stupid older brother who I've known since he rode a tricycle? As *if!* What are you thinking? That is the stupidest thing ever. When did you two start hatching this stupid idea?" She threw her books and magazines to the floor and slid further beneath the covers. "I get sick and what do my friends do?" she muttered. "Start stupid rumors behind my back." She paused to gather what little strength she had and then used it up, yelling, "*I do not like Michael Malcolm MacGillivray!*"

Amy blinked, silenced, but only for a moment. "Well, okaaaaay, then! Point taken! Fine!"

"Fine!" Jane yelled.

"Fine!" Amy hollered.

Flory kept her eyes trained on Minnie as she scratched the space between her ears and the small white ruff under her chin.

Jane lay back on the pillows, exhausted, and closed her eyes. Flory began to think maybe she'd fallen asleep, and signaled Amy to leave the room, when suddenly she spoke. "Tell me about your fabulous jobs again," she said, a small smile on her face. "Ame, you first. No, wait, you first, Flory. And slow down when you get to the part about Rand Harbinsale's face."

Mike leaned over, keeping one hand on the wheel and taking Katrina's hand in the other, and did another circuit of the Cedar's Ridge Senior Secondary School grounds. The rental car, his suit, and Katrina's corsage had cost him two weeks' wages, but the way he figured, you only graduate once. This was it, and they were going to do it right. Katrina looked like a movie starlet in a curve-hugging, full-length red dress, blond hair piled high, just a few wisps framing her face. He was looking forward to brushing those wisps aside with his fingers each time he kissed her. And if he did say so himself, he looked pretty not-so-bad, either. Black suit, crisp white shirt, black tie. She'd bought him a red rose for his boutonniere, so they matched. Perfectly.

A warm June breeze caused the maples and poplars surrounding the school to sway and bow like courtiers as the shiny black convertible made its grand tour. Couples and small groups were piling out of limousines and vintage cars of every size and color, the boys slowly losing their awkwardness in their formal clothes and the girls' dresses sparkling like jewels in the warm glow of the setting sun. Friends waved, and Mike and Katrina waved back, smiling and laughing. "This must be what it feels like to be royalty!" Katrina exclaimed as they looped down below the soccer field. "I could get used to this, Mooky! Couldn't you?"

"What's that, Kat," he teased, "don't want to be a farmer's wife?" She burst out laughing and didn't deign to answer.

Mike nodded, keeping his eyes on the road. It was a perfect evening, and even their running "discussion" about his future—their future—couldn't distract him tonight. It was summer, the air was warm, and the sky was a riot of blues and pinks. There would be stars later. And he was graduating. The thought made him elated and anxious all at once. He still hadn't settled on what he would do come September. Kat was sure she knew. As for him, he'd never been less sure of anything in his life. But tonight was all sewn up. It was his grad night. He could forget about everything else for now.

Katrina's cell phone rang in her purse. "Kat! Tonight of all nights. I thought you were going to leave that thing at home!" He spoke teasingly, but inside he felt a little pang of annoyance. She'd promised. She spent practically all her time between classes and after school calling and text-messaging friends, and he didn't mind all that much. Most people did the same. But this was grad night . . .

"Oh, Mooks, never mind," she simpered, trying to placate him. "It's probably just Leila or Chiclet wondering where we are. I *did* tell them we'd be inside by now . . . Hello, hey, this is Kat . . ."

"Oh, hey! What's up? Yeah, right beside me, I'll put him on, okay?" She held out the phone, sighing. "It's your little sister, Mike."

"Ame? Everything okay?" Spotting a place to pull over, he shut off the engine. He listened for several seconds, feeling his throat constrict and his heart grow tight in his chest. Then, "Mom and dad have already left for the lake? No, no, I know you wouldn't ask tonight if you didn't have to. I'll be right there." He flipped the phone shut, passed it back to Katrina, and started the car all in one fluid move.

"What's up, Mooky?" Kat asked, her eyes narrowing with suspicion. "You'll be right *where*?"

"It's Buster," he answered, struggling for control of his voice. Whipping the convertible around in a screeching U-turn, he stepped on the gas and made to exit the school grounds.

"Wait a minute . . . your dog? We're leaving because of your dog? What's the plan, Mooks—to miss our graduation?" Katrina spoke quietly, but Mike was pretty sure this was the calm before the proverbial storm.

Buster had started vomiting earlier in the week and graduated to a particularly nasty case of diarrhea that had kept them all running for the carpet stain remover. At first, they'd assumed he'd eaten a tennis ball or a shoe or some hapless dead squirrel he'd found in the trails and was suffering from indigestion. But when the situation failed to improve on its own, the MacGillivrays rushed him up the hill to Dr. Reid. The old neighborhood vet had been caring for Buster since he was a pup—since Mike himself was just eight years old, he realized, the lump in his throat growing larger—and was intimately familiar with the retriever's eclectic tastes in snacks. Dr. Reid examined him and gave him IV fluids, took X-rays, sent some blood work to the lab, and kept him overnight. He told the MacGillivrays to monitor him carefully over the next few days. Since then, Buster hadn't seemed much better, but he hadn't gotten worse, either. Not until tonight.

"Amy says he's stumbling and shaking," Mike answered now, still shaken himself by the panic in his sister's voice. "Can't walk properly or control his legs. It's bad, Kat. My mom and dad have gone to Cultus and Amy's home alone with him without a car. Somebody's got to get him to emergency."

"And that somebody has to be you, I suppose? Responsible, reliable older brother saves the day? C'mon, Mike, not tonight. This is your grad. *Our* grad. Amy's a big girl. She can take care of the dog." Katrina's voice was still calm, but tinged with reproach. "Here, call her back, here's the number for a taxi. Mooky, it's grad!" She held out her cell phone.

He hesitated for just a second, but then shook his head. "Buster's my dog, Kat. My . . . he's my friend. Since forever. I don't know what's wrong with him, but I'm not sending him to the emergency clinic in a taxi. I . . . I'd like you to come with me. I'll understand, of course, if you don't want to. But I've got to go." He pulled the convertible up to the school entrance and let the car idle.

"Oh. My. God." Katrina sat perfectly still, staring down at her sparkly gold shoes, tendrils of hair falling across her face. Mike wanted desperately to touch her, but he didn't dare. "I cannot believe you're asking me to take off this dress before I've even had a chance to dance in it!"

Mike looked over at her miserably, only to find her staring back at him with a wicked grin on her face. His eyes widened in surprise. He'd been sure he'd lost her. Was it possible he was going to miss his grad and still be the luckiest grade twelve guy at Cedar's Ridge High?

He grasped Kat's face in his hands and kissed her long and hard. "You don't have to take your dress off," he whispered against her neck. He couldn't bear to see her in sweats just yet, not after all the time he'd spent anticipating this night. "You'll be the belle of the . . . of the veterinary hospital, Kat. Don't take it off."

She pulled away slightly, a question in her eyes. "Ever?"

He held her away from him then, hoping he hadn't misunderstood. "Well, not yet, anyway." His voice cracked. She grinned again, and he held her gaze for as long as he could stand it, then he kissed her again.

"Thanks, Kat," he said gruffly.

"Hmph," was her answer. "And you say *I'm* high maintenance!" He laughed and pulled her closer. "Um, Mike?" She spoke in a whisper against his ear.

"Yeah?" he answered hoarsely.

"Isn't this an emergency?"

There was a pause. "Oh my god, *Buster*!" He pulled himself free, spun the car around, and raced for home.

22

THE MESSENGER AND THE MESSAGE

JANE KNEW FOR SURE she'd kicked the flu bug, if only because the walk through the gauntlet didn't kill her. It was the last Thursday in June—summer was officially a week old—and between heat that made the air ripple and protestors that made it resound with jeers, Jane arrived at the UWRC sweat-soaked and shaking. "If the global warming doesn't get you, the warm welcome will," she muttered to herself.

She yanked open the door and stepped inside to find Anthony at the reception desk singing "God Save the Queen," his shock of long black bangs swinging to and fro in time to the marching tune. In spite of herself, she laughed. "What's the occasion, Anthony? Is Her Royal Highness dropping by later today? Maybe with a small donation?"

"Nice!" He gave her a high-five, laughing now, too. "Hey, Jane-girl, you ever seen the changing of the guard at Buckingham Palace?" She shook her head. "The guys in red with the big poofy hats? Great hats, I must say. Anyhoo, the old guys march away, the new guys march in, boom, done. And unless you look reeeeeeeal close, you'd never know the difference." He waved a hand casually toward the door, the eloquent gesture encompassing at once the mass of protestors and their impact on the wildlife center over the past three weeks. "Same," he concluded simply. "Minus the hats."

Jane narrowed her eyes. She'd kept her head down this morning, ignoring the signs, tuning out the shouts. "Anthony, are you saying this is a *different* bunch of people from the ones who were threatening us a couple of weeks ago? That there's *more* people who want us dead than we thought? Because if that's what you're saying, then I'm really not sure why you're singing."

"It's what I'm saying, girlfriend," he responded. "Yesterday, the Board issued a news release announcing that they are rescinding the euthanasia policy with respect to crows."

Jane's jaw dropped. "After everything everybody's been through?"

"*Because* of everything everybody's been through," Anthony replied. "They can't stand the pressure any more, and they don't think the staff and volunteers should have to, either." He forced a grin. "Nobody blames them, really. Call them crazy, but they don't want to see a building get torched or a volunteer get lynched. Righty-o? Bottom line, though, they're doing it to save the Center. Donations have dropped off so bad that they're looking at letting the summer staff go.

Whoops! I probably wasn't supposed to mention that to you." Jane shrugged, unable to feel sorry for herself in the midst of such news. Maybe she was just numb, but her summer job seemed a small concern next to the survival of the Center.

Anthony continued, "The freezers have been empty since last week, and we're feeding the patients with whatever the local grocers will donate at the end of each day—the ones who aren't boycotting us, that is. It came down to 'change the policy or die.' So effective next Tuesday, right after the long weekend, the policy's gone."

Jane struggled to absorb the news. She'd always known the Center operated on a shoestring budget and the goodwill of their volunteers and donors. But she'd also always taken it for granted that it could continue to do so indefinitely. Now its very survival was threatened. And if the Center didn't survive, neither would the thousands of animals it took in every year.

She pointed to the door behind her: "And the protestors?"

"Up until yesterday, it was animal rights extremists who couldn't see the wisdom of euthanizing crows brought to the Center in order to save the lives of the majority of our patients—and possibly our staff and volunteers as well." It was Evie who answered. She'd arrived at the reception area smelling of detergent and bleach, a load of wet towels in her arms.

"Today, it's the pest-people, as I call them. Everybody from pesticide-happy homeowners who have no idea how much their green lawns cost the ecosystem they're a part of, all the way up to types like our crow murderer from last month, who'd be happiest if we could find a way to exterminate every crow in Cedar's Ridge. They're furious that the Board is withdrawing the policy, and feel we're putting the entire city in danger of contracting West Nile Virus by doing so. They're picketing our suppliers and even the airports, trying to cut us off from food and medical supplies in the hope that it'll convince us to stop treating crows. They consider them pests, along with a whole host of other sentient creatures—not worthy of treatment at all."

Evie sighed heavily, worn with worry and fatigue. "There's so much misinformation and misunderstanding out there, and I'm afraid every time we make a new decision here, we're just adding to the confusion."

"I agree with Anthony, though," Evie continued. "The Board's not the culprit here, any more than the staff were for recommending the policy in the first place. The real danger is West Nile Virus, and if it does arrive this summer, as predicted, and we're accepting crows, as we will be again as of next Tuesday, it will decimate our patients. Without the vaccine, which we can't afford, without quarantine facilities, without surplus food, medications, caging, even laundry supplies for the additional patient load, without extra staff and additional volunteers, there is no way the Center will survive the onslaught of this disease. There are older volunteers who are afraid they won't survive it either. You'll notice Avis isn't here today. I don't expect to see her back until October." Her expression was bleak. Anthony stared down at the reception desk. Jane's mind reeled.

"With the policy in place, we lose our donors and shut our doors. Without it, we lose our patients—our reason for being—and shut our doors. Either way you slice it, it looks like this could be the UWRC's last summer." Evie turned to head outside to the drying lines.

Without considering what she was asking, what she might be offering, Jane blurted, "So what do we do?"

"For today," Evie responded, giving her a direct look, "it's business as usual. Jane, would you please assist Daniel on meds?"

Jane had learned over time to decipher the hiero-glyphics that covered the meds board: an animal's case number, type and quantity of medication, whether it was administered once a day or twice, in the morning or the evening. Daniel had already drawn up the syringes filled with antibiotics to fight infections, and steroids to reduce swelling in animals with central nervous system damage; ointments for eye injuries and skin abrasions; bandages for wrapping wounds or making splints; mineral oil to counteract StickiStep; charcoal to bind to poisons and help eliminate them from an animal's system. *The pest people have been busy,* she thought grimly.

The meds were grouped together and lined up on the exam room counter in the order that each animal appeared on the board. One by one, Jane retrieved the patients from the care room, weighed them to ensure they were eating well, and then assisted Daniel in administering their medications. They worked well together, without much need for talk. Occasionally, Daniel would demonstrate a new technique for wrapping an injured wing, or for extending the neck of a bird during tube-feeding to ensure the patient didn't regurgitate its meal. She'd learned much from him over the months, and especially enjoyed these shifts working hands-on with the neediest of their patients.

Wilson's Warbler; young female; bright gold and tinged with green; about four inches long; weight on arrival 18.5 g; seen hitting window; CNS damage likely. Rx: 0.01 cc steroid BID, standard caging, no heat, no perch, standard diet.

Jane checked the level in the syringe against the prescribed amount, then moved in close to inject the little bird with the steroid while Daniel held it still on the exam table, head covered to reduce stress, breast exposed. Blowing gently on the breast feathers to reveal the keel, Jane measured a quarter inch out from the bone and injected the steroid into the tissues just beneath the skin. Withdrawing the needle, she applied slight pressure to the injection site to prevent bruising, then disposed of the needle in the hazards box as Daniel rewrapped the patient for return to its cage.

"Nice work, Jane!" Katrina's voice just behind her shoulder startled her. Jane hadn't even heard her come into the exam room. "Hey, Daniel, does this raccoon diet look okay to you?"

Daniel threw a glance across the examining table before turning his attention back to the meds board. "That robin with the wing wrap is up next, Jane. Yeah, Kat, perfect. No need to check with me. You know your stuff."

"Oh, I know. I just wanted to make sure you *liked* my stuff!" Katrina winked and flounced out of the room, blond ponytail flying behind her.

Was she just flirting? Jane thought furiously. *She was flirting! Katrina D'Angelo, spoken-for girlfriend of Mike MacGillivray, was flirting with Daniel!* She hurried down the hall to retrieve the injured robin and to accidentally on purpose run into Katrina.

"So Kat," she said in what she hoped was a casual tone, her back to the care room as she scooped the robin from its cage, "how was grad?"

"Oh, pffft," Katrina made a derisive sound, "what a gong show. I spent the night in the hospital."

"What?" Jane cried. Katrina looked okay. Was it Mike? "What happened?"

Katrina waved a hand dismissively. "I figured you'd know . . . you know, from Amy. Let's just say grad night wasn't what I'd had in mind, okay? The family dog had some kind of major freak-out and *my* boyfriend had to save the day! So we spent grad at the 24-hour vet clinic. With his *sister*. Til, like, six in the morning." She sighed, picking up a tray of dirty dishes. "I love animals, right, but seriously, between grad and that university info session thing and now with Mike leaving for the farm for the summer, I am really having trouble feeling like number one on that boy's to-do list." She turned toward the kitchen.

"Wait . . . but, so how's Buster?" Jane's stomach was knotted and her mouth was dry. Amy had told her on Saturday that Buster had been sick, but clearly he'd worsened. And she hadn't so much as checked in with her friend to get the news.

"Oh! Fine, now," Katrina answered as she left the care room. "Alive, anyway. Did Amy not tell you any of this? I thought you two told each other everything!"

"I've been . . . she probably didn't want to worry me," Jane answered miserably, though Katrina was already gone.

More than ever, Jane was glad Daniel was more action than talk. She needed time to think, to sort through everything she'd heard—from Anthony, from Evie, from Katrina. She had greatly missed Avis's pragmatic cantankerousness over the past weeks, and wondered how she'd get through the rest of the summer without her. *If* she still had a job at all by next week. *If* the Center was still running.

By 11:30, they'd reached the last notation on the board: three baby squirrels, grays, found abandoned in a box on the sidewalk outside the mall. Daniel had fed them first thing that morning. It was her turn. She found the squirrels, one black, one a dark brindled gray, and one a light gray-brown, knotted together in a somnambulant ball in their flannel-lined cage. "You first," she whispered to the black, extracting the tiny, mewling handful from the pile.

By ten minutes to noon, the black and brindled were fed and asleep again in their cage, and she sat on a stool in the exam room, the runty gray wrapped in a soft cloth in her lap, elated as she watched him finally grasp the feeding syringe between his front paws and suck.

There came a tapping behind her at the exam room window. Jane ignored it—just a branch moving in the breeze. There it was again, though, a steady "tap tap tap," and it occurred to her suddenly that there *was* no breeze today. And then she recognized the sound, remembered it from that morning at Cultus. She turned on her stool, knowing who she'd see. It was Crow.

"Daniel!" she called urgently. "*Daniel!*"

He arrived running, his face white. Too many things

had gone wrong in the past weeks not to take a call for help extremely seriously. "What is it, Jane? Are you okay? What's wrong?" He looked wildly around the room. Then he, too, spotted the crow at the window. Tap, tap, tap. "What the . . . ?"

"Daniel, it's Crow!" Jane said, still sheltering the squirrel in her arms.

"Uh, I can see that." The color was beginning to return to his face. "Jane, please tell me you didn't cry wolf because of a crow?" His voice was even, but Jane knew that if she didn't explain fast, the tension would take its toll.

"No," she said firmly. "Not because of *any* crow. Daniel, I know this crow. I'm sure that sounds crazy, but she belongs to someone, someone I know." She paused, as a thought struck her: "The only reason I can think of for her to come all the way here from Cultus Lake is that she's got a message for us. See that band on her leg?"

Crow was scrabbling at the sill, trying to find purchase on the narrow ledge. Daniel narrowed his eyes and then nodded. "Well, I'll be . . . Do you think she'll let us catch her? She looks exhausted, not surprising if she's flown from the Fraser Valley! I'll get a net."

"Here!" Jane passed the wrapped squirrel to a surprised Daniel and, stepping forward, unlatched the window and slid it open. The shouts and chanting of the protestors hit her like a wall, but her attention was on Crow. Would the bird remember her? Trust her? Surely she was the reason the animal was here?

Yes. Pushing off from the sill, Crow rose slightly into the air and then blew into the room like a feather, settling herself on the examining table in front of Jane. She was, as Daniel had said, exhausted. Hot, panting, head lolling forward, eyelids drooping, tail feathers sagging. It was high noon on the hottest day of the year so far, and this seventeen-plus-year-old bird had just flown over sixty miles, homing in somehow on a destination she'd never seen.

Daniel had gently placed the wrapped and dozing squirrel in a kennel on a heating pad, and was donning gloves. He tossed a second pair to Jane. "Masks, too," he said, handing her one. "And close that window and pull the blinds and hope nobody out there saw what just happened. If we're lucky, we can get away with pretending she came in next Tuesday, and you did *not* hear me say that and I swear I'll deny it if you ever bring it up."

Jane felt her throat tighten and tears sting behind her eyes. It could have been because of Daniel's willingness to break all the rules to save Crow. Or it could have been because it was too late. As she watched, gray-black lids closed over small, shiny brown domes, mischief and wisdom extinguished.

"I'm so sorry, Jane," Daniel said softly. He reached for the heavy, sealable plastic bags and then hesitated, not sure whether Jane was ready.

"Not yet," she returned, holding up a hand. "There's still the message." She'd laid Crow gently on the soft towel that covered the exam table, and now she reached for the band that circled her left leg and clicked it open, withdrawing a narrow, ragged scrap of paper.

Block letters, pencil, a shaky hand, but a hand she knew, she was sure.

I AM THE MESSENGER AND THE MESSAGE WHERE YOU LOOK FOR HER YOU WILL NOT FIND HER

Daniel made a slight noise from over her shoulder. "I . . . I don't understand. Shouldn't it say, 'and the message *is,* where you look for her you will not find her'? Isn't there a word missing? Although even if there is, I still don't get it. Do you, Jane? Do you know what it means?"

Crow flies the course between the spirit world and the earth walk, carrying messages from the living to the dead, and from the dead to the living. No, all the words were there. *I am the messenger and the message.* Jane understood perfectly. The Crone—Audrey—was dead.

Daniel left her on her own to say her goodbyes and to finish the procedure of preparing Crow for delivery to the provincial lab for testing. Double-seal in two heavy plastic bags and refrigerate until delivery. Practical, respectful, impersonal. The familiar, ritual-like actions helped calm her.

Jane checked the schedule. No delivery until next Wednesday. That was a long time to wait, and this message was urgent. Poking her head into the reception area, Jane found Anthony's chair empty. He'd gone for lunch and left the phones on auto-answer. Glancing quickly down the hall, she checked her watch—just past noon, they'd be in the cafeteria—then picked up the receiver and quickly punched in Flory's cell phone number.

"Flor, hi!" She spoke fast and in a half-whisper. "Sorry for using up daytime minutes. Is Amy there with you? It's important. Thanks. Hey, Ame, I gotta make this quick: I have a crow here that needs to jump the testing queue at the lab. Is there any way you could convince somebody there to make that happen? Like, today? No, I wouldn't be asking for just any crow." Her voice wobbled. "It's Crow. Audrey's Crow." She listened as Amy reacted, then told Flory the news. "So? Can you do it? I can pick you up outside the caf in ten minutes. We'll be back before the one o'clock bell. Thanks, Ame. No, you won't get fired. Thanks. Bye."

Returning to the exam room, she took up the tightly sealed bundle and wrapped it in towels, then stowed it in her backpack. *Time for a new backpack anyway*, she thought. Then she said goodbye to Evie and Daniel, stepped outside and into the fray, and ran her second eight-minute mile of the day.

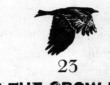

23
AS THE CROW FLIES

EVIE JORDAN CLOSED THE DOOR of the Urban Wildlife Rescue Center behind her, weary to the bone. *Every time I lock that door from now on, I'm going to wonder whether it's for the last time,* she thought. It was Friday night, just after 8:00 p.m. A dusky blue-orange light filtered through the trees in the garden, and the baby birds, indoors and out, were finally asleep for the night. Despite the extended summer hours, diehard protestors still lined the access road well into the evenings, and the walk back to her car was no more pleasant than the walk to the Center in the mornings. She'd actually given up wondering when she'd ever be able to drive all the way to work again.

Checking the address she'd scrawled on the scrap of paper once again, she wondered whether she'd be able to drive straight there, or whether she'd have to kick Plan B into gear. Glancing in the rear-view mirror as she pulled away, she saw four other cars spew sudden gusts of exhaust as they started to roll. Ah. Plan B, then.

They'd been following her home, picketing the

street she lived on, sticking signs into her lawn, calling her by name. She hated that the most, that familiarity, that pretended intimacy from people who knew her not at all, understood her not at all. They. Them. Who were they, anyway? These animal lovers? These pest warriors? People with lives and jobs and families and dogs, just like her. Standing up for what they believed in. Just like her. *Viva democracy,* she thought wryly. *And viva the free press while we're at it.* They'd had letters, more than a handful, from thoughtful people who agreed with the UWRC's decisions and wanted to show their support. Some even enclosed cheques. But although she'd forwarded copies to the media, none had made the news. *If no news is good news,* she thought, *then good news is no news. Bad news sells. And we're all about the bottom line. All of us,* she thought bitterly, the truth hitting her once again that that's what it had come to for the wildlife hospital as well.

By the time she left the access road and hit the main street, the four cars on her tail had become seven. A proper caravan. *Well, I'm not going home just yet,* she said aloud to her side mirror, *so let's have a little fun!* She hit the gas and took a sharp right at the next corner, then wound through the back roads, left, then right, then right again, until she counted only three cars behind her. *And now I need a little distance,* she whispered. *May the speeding ticket gods be with me tonight!*

Careening around the next corner, she looped back

along the main street, gunning it to get through the amber light. *I am so bad,* she chastised herself, feeling better than she had in weeks. *But this is so much fun!* She glanced in the mirror. She'd put some distance between them, but her pursuers were still there. *Fun, yet frightening,* she corrected, a shot of adrenaline bursting into her bloodstream. At the next light, she took a sharp right, peeled along the quiet residential street, scanning frantically for cats and small children, then right again at the next intersection. Down the hill, no need for brakes, til she could see Elfin Lake below and to her left. A squealing left at the bottom of the hill, into the parking lot of the little lakeshore park, and there, last spot, closest to the boat rentals.

Backpack on, doors locked. Quick check: nobody behind her. Yet. She threw herself at the rentals counter: "One rowboat, please," she gasped. *All small crafts must be safely docked no later than 9:00 p.m., or patrons will be charged the full day rate,* the sign read. A quick glance at her watch: 8:35. Not in a million years. "Do you have an overnight rate?" she asked the teenage boy behind the counter.

He grinned and winked at her. "Who's the lucky guy?"

"Oh, for . . . here!" Evie slapped down a twenty, grabbed the oars out of his hands and tore to the dock. She could hear the caravan now. They'd arrived at the lake. They'd see her leave in the boat. Would they actually follow her out onto the water? *Ah, well, that's what we came up with Plan B for,* she reminded herself, stepping tipsily into the rowboat. Within seconds, she'd stowed her bag under the hard wooden seat and sculled away from the dock.

If it weren't for the fact that I'm being pursued by crazy people, this would be quite charming! she thought, taking a moment to get her bearings. The sun still lit the western sky behind her with tufts of pink and gold, and the moon was rising before her eyes against a backdrop of indigo. A night for artists and lovers.

And crazy people. She glanced back over her left shoulder. She could just make out the old farmhouse, set well back from the shore, but once she'd found it, she easily spotted the white fence and the little boat dock at its terminus. That was her destination. She altered her course slightly and pulled.

Hearing the slap of oars, she turned back quickly to find that her pursuers had, indeed, rented boats of their own. Unbelievable! Her heart was pounding now, and not only from the exertion of rowing. Just what did they plan to do? They couldn't hope to get away with anything drastic . . . could they? It was just scare tactics, that's all.

That's all. *Oh, heaven,* she thought, *that was enough. Enough to exhaust them all and leave them afraid to come to work, afraid to go home. Enough to divide them, pit them against one another, cause fights and bitter accusations and resignations. Enough to close the Center forever.*

The little dock was in sight now. *Please please please let this be the right one,* she prayed as she brought herself alongside with trembling arms. There was no one on the dock or in the yard, or waiting by the door. But there. There was a winking in the upstairs window. It came again, like the reflection of moonlight in a child's hand mirror. She'd arrived. She tied the boat securely and, with one last glance at her pursuers, ran up the path.

Mrs. MacGillivray let her into the darkened foyer and closed the front door quickly before introducing herself and giving her a warm hug. Evie hadn't realized how much she'd needed one until that moment. Clearing her throat, she smiled gratefully at this woman who'd just adopted her. "Very cloak and dagger, hey?" she joked. Mrs. MacGillivray drew the curtain aside slightly and glanced out at the lake.

"Very," she replied, entirely serious. "Let me take you to the girls now." She led Evie downstairs and through the basement, picking up a pair of flashlights en route. At the eastern bearing wall, she stopped in front of a low wooden door. "This opens into a passageway that runs under the ground to the Shack . . . er, to where the girls are. You're not claustrophobic, are you, Evelyn?" Evie shook her head, lips pressed tight together. *Not tonight, anyway.* She took a deep breath and followed Mrs. MacGillivray into the passage.

The way through was black, narrow, and low. Crouching, she kept the flashlight's wan beam trained on Mrs. MacGillivray's white tennis shoes. At some point, she lost count of her steps and started again. It was the only thing that kept her from spinning on her heel and running screaming from the tunnel.

At last, the feet in the spotlight stopped moving, and she heard Mrs. MacGillivray knock on something wooden above and ahead of them. There was a squeal of rusty hinges, and then light, and air. Oh, blessed air. She realized a set of crudely made steps rose up directly in front of her, and she climbed them to find herself inside the infamous Shack.

"I'll leave you four alone," said Mrs. MacGillivray, turning to descend into the passage once again. "Malcolm and I are waiting to hear from the vet. Goodnight, Evelyn. And good luck."

The small room was silent except for the quiet hum of the computer. No soft whumping of Buster's tail on the floor—he was in the hospital again after a relapse of his baffling illness. Mysterious shadows danced around them, made by candlelight as it sought out the objects in Amy's laboratory and projected them, larger than life, on the walls and ceiling. Jane, Amy, and Flory sat around the rickety old table in the center of the room, and all three looked up expectantly at Evie. She pulled out the fourth chair and joined them at the table.

"So," Jane began, her expression serious, "any

trouble getting here?" It was after 9:00 p.m. now. They'd been waiting for Evie since 8:00. The Center was less than half a mile away. There'd been trouble, there was no doubt of that.

"None whatsoever," was Evie's equally serious reply. Then her face broke into an enormous grin, and the three friends were shaking with suppressed laughter. "Oh, girls, you have no idea!" she said, and launched into an energetic retelling of her narrow escape.

As she wound down, Evie sat back in her chair and folded her arms. "And now, Ms. Ray, would you care to tell me exactly what I've been dodging bullets *for*? Your invitation to this lovely soirée was more than a little cryptic."

Jane cleared her throat, glancing quickly at Amy and Flory. "Right," she said. "It's about what you said at the meeting yesterday, about how the UWRC suddenly has money but no way to spend it on what we need. Well . . . we think we can spend it for you."

Evie had called an emergency staff meeting at 4:00 p.m. Thursday afternoon, and had included Jane as a courtesy, since she wouldn't officially be starting work until the following week. They'd gathered in the exam room with the door closed, the sun beating in through the western window, electric pads radiating heat under the new admissions, the air stifling with tension and expectation.

"The UWRC has just received notice of an unexpected bequest," Evie began in her usual abrupt way.

"A large one. Enough to purchase vaccination dosages to last us through mosquito season." There were gasps all around and tentative smiles as the staff looked at one another with hope for the first time in weeks. Evie's face remained impassive. She continued: "I put word out to the national rehabbers' network this afternoon as soon as I heard the news about the donation. Rocky Mountain Wildlife Hospital in Alberta thinks they can get us the quantities we need." She paused. "Then I started calling shippers." She paused again, and looked at the floor. "No one'll touch us."

"We've been on the national news for weeks now," she pressed on, "and not in a good light. We're a political hot potato, and nobody wants to get burned. I heard every excuse in the book, but the bottom line is, nobody will deliver the vaccine."

"Send me to Alberta, Evie," Daniel broke in. "I'll smuggle it back in a carry-on or something. It's craziness that we're so close to . . . we can't let a couple of courier companies stand in our way!"

Evie nodded. "Thanks, Dan. I thought you might offer. But even if we all decided that an airline ticket for you was a justifiable use of this donation, you'd never get off the ground. Think about it! You've been tailed to and from work every day for weeks, just like I have! They know your face, your vehicle, your schedule. You'd be mobbed at the airport, and I'm afraid of what a crowd like that might do. To their way of thinking, crows are a threat to public health, and more than that, vermin—something to exterminate, not rehabilitate . . . never mind vaccinate!" She shook her head. "It's way too dangerous. And besides, I need you here. I can't carry this place alone."

Daniel nodded and bowed his head. Beth echoed his offer, and Evie turned her down, too, for all the same reasons. "The Board is waiting to hear from me, and I've decided on the course of action I plan to recommend. With your agreement, of course," she added belatedly. The still, stuffy room was silent. All of them listened. This was Evie's decision and they knew it. But they appreciated being included in it, and they trusted she'd hear them out if they had anything to add. Evie gazed around at each of them. Jane noted again how worn she looked, beaten down by the events of the past weeks. She hoped against hope that what Evie was about to say was brilliant, creative, the perfect solution. But how could it be? The head staffer had no energy left for brilliant solutions. Everything in her was geared now to mere survival.

"We hunker down," Evie began. "Do whatever it takes to get through the season with minimal losses. Convince the Board to keep the doors open, even if we have to do it with a skeleton crew." *Good grief,* Jane thought, looking around at the little group. *How much more skeletal could they get?* "And then we put the money toward vaccines for next year, when things have died down," Evie was saying, "spend the fall and winter raising money for a quarantine facility, use the spring to build it." She shrugged, a defeated gesture. "The vaccine by itself won't save our butts anyway, even if we *could* get our hands on it for this summer. Better to look ahead, to the future. This situation won't last forever. It can't." Jane heard the unspoken question: *Can it?*

Evie gazed around again at her crew. She was looking *for* something, Jane thought, something specific, in a face, a pair of eyes. What? Agreement? Support? No, she realized suddenly. Evie was looking for a better idea. And none of them had one.

Slowly, they nodded, understanding that this was the proposal she would put to the Board, this was the law they'd live by—or die by—this summer. Jane wondered whether any of the others had heard Evie's unspoken plea for a better alternative, and doubted it. They were *all* exhausted, too much so to be reading between lines or thinking outside the proverbial box.

"Evie," she asked quietly as the others shuffled slowly out of the room, "may I ask who made the bequest?" If her guess was right, then she'd know for sure not to give up, that there had to be a way to get the medicine to the crows and the other animals this year.

"Somebody from the Valley," Evie replied, closing her eyes and frowning in concentration. "A-something. Alice, maybe? Ainsley?"

"Audrey?"

"That's it, yes. Audrey. A Mrs. Audrey Thomas. Her whole life savings, by the looks of it. Such a gift." She turned and headed down the hallway, and Jane barely caught her last words: "Such a waste."

And so Jane had taken the conundrum back to Amy and Flory, fresh minds, unspoiled by proximity to the protests and the infighting and the death threats. And together, the three of them had found their way out of the box and into a brand new idea. Once hatched, they mulled over it and reworked it and made notes and calculations, and finally, well into the wee hours, they decided it was good. Whereupon Jane had called Evie, and invited her to join them Friday evening. It had taken some convincing, but she'd done it. And Evie had made it. Just. Now to make her fall in love with their plan.

"I'll go," Jane said. "That is, we'll go," she amended, nodding at her two best friends before turning back to gauge Evie's reaction. "We'll take my car. No one will recognize it. Heck, it's been so long since I washed it that it's not even the same color it was last month! We'll slip out of town, completely unnoticed, pick up the vaccine from the Rocky Mountain Wildlife folks, and be back by Monday afternoon, just in time for Tuesday when the policy reversal goes into effect!" She grinned at Evie, triumphant. The plan was flawless.

"Let me get this straight," Evie wasn't smiling. In fact, she sounded angry. "You three propose to drive straight from Cedar's Ridge to Alberta by yourselves, paying for the gas with, what, your weekly allowances? And at the same time manage to outrun the good folks on both sides of this issue who'd happily see us wildlife rescue types dead?" She shook her head and laughed, grimly. "Not a chance, girls. It's way too dangerous, and for that matter, way too insane. I said no to my other staff. I'm saying no to you." She looked pointedly at Jane, daring her to argue.

Jane met her gaze, surprised by how calm she felt. She had absolutely no doubt about what Audrey's money was for, why she'd left it to the UWRC. *Not* to be put in a bank account and saved for next summer, of that she was certain. Next summer would be too late. It was for right now. "Until next Tuesday," she responded, her voice steady, "I'm a volunteer, not an employee of the UWRC. And I volunteer to go."

Amy and Flory pulled bulging backpacks out from under the table and held them up in the candle light. "Us, too," they added in unison.

"And it would be a shame," Jane continued, still surprised by the sound of her own voice, "if we arrived at Rocky Mountain only to find that the money hadn't been wired for the vaccine, and we had to come home empty-handed."

Evie groaned and put her head in her hands. "This is crazy! I can't let you do this."

"Evie," Jane said softly, "don't you see? You have to!

Your plan won't work. The Center will be closed by fall and you know it. This is our only chance."

"Evie," Amy jumped in, "if I may say, with all due respect, it's just a road trip. You know, the kind of thing young foolish teenagers like us do all the time in the summer!"

Flory took a turn. "It seems big to you—it *is* big to you," she said gently, "because you're so close to it. To us, it really is just a fun way to start our summer vacation. Please, Evie?"

"But how will you pay for the gas? Which route will you take? Are you sure it's even possible to get back on time?" Evie looked round the little gathering, eyes questioning, then she clapped a hand to her forehead, realizing what she'd done. She'd just spoken as though they were really going to do this. They'd heard it, too, and let out muffled whoops.

Flory promptly pulled out a black file folder she'd kept hidden under the table and laid out the notes and calculations they'd made—the various possible routes over the mountains, the mileage, ETAs there and back. For the next fifteen minutes, the four of them pored over the file, discussing every detail, arguing over the map, debating the merits and drawbacks of each route.

"Flor," Jane said suddenly, "can you bring up a more detailed map on the computer?" Flory went at once to the desk and attacked the keyboard. "Ame, Evie's right about gas money. It's way more than we calculated.

Do you think your mom and dad might . . . ?" She left the question hanging. She hated to ask, but she knew she couldn't ask her own parents, not right now, when they were just climbing out of the red with the restaurant. Maybe Flory's uncles at the law firm . . . ?

"Jane, I think we can eliminate all possible routes but one—this one." Flory gestured for them to join her at the computer and pointed to a thin yellow line running east-west across the screen. "You've been following crows since that rescue back in May, haven't you?" Jane nodded, grudgingly. She had to admit, one crow had led to another . . . and another and another. For better or for worse. "Well," Flory's voice was rising with excitement, "why stop now?"

They peered over Flory's shoulder at the screen. Jane gasped when she saw the route her friend had mapped out: Highway 3 east through Hope, Osoyoos, and Creston leading to Crowsnest Provincial Park, past the Crowfoot Glacier, and on to the Municipality of Crowsnest Pass, where it was just a short drive to Rocky Mountain Wildlife Hospital. "And all beneath the invisible eye of the Corvus constellation!" Flory breathed.

Amy shook her head, flabbergasted. "And now, ladies and gentleman, the same magical faerie that just planned our itinerary for us will suddenly sprinkle money down from the stars to pay for . . ."

The red phone on the desk rang like a fire alarm, startling them all. Flory screamed, then clapped a hand to her mouth. Amy recovered first and lifted the receiver.

"Hello? I'm sorry, who? Oh! Oh, yes! We met last fall. Of course. Very nice to hear from you, ma'am." The other three exchanged bewildered looks. Who on earth was calling the Shack at 9:30 at night? "Yes, as a matter of fact, she's right here. Just hold the line a moment, please." Amy held the phone out to Jane: "It's your friend Avis."

Jane's eyes went wide. She hadn't seen or heard from Avis for weeks. Hadn't thought to call her, either, she realized now, feeling ashamed. The truth was, she'd been angry with her for staying away from the Center. Logically, she knew the mile walk through jeering protestors was too much for anyone of her age, but somehow she'd still expected her friend to be there each week. Belatedly, she realized she'd let the protestors win by dividing them. She'd been disloyal to her friend. What on earth would she say to her *now?* She took the receiver from Amy. "Uh, hello?"

"Jane, this is Avis," the older woman said unnecessarily. "Edna on the UWRC Board called me this afternoon and told me everything. It was your friend from the trailer park, wasn't it? The donor? Yes, I thought I recalled the name. And then Evie called to ask if I knew what you were 'up to,' that was the phrase she used, 'up to.' And I said no, I hadn't spoken to you in some time." Jane winced. "So I spent my supper hour thinking about it and put two and two together and thought, my missy will be over those mountains before you can say 'Jack Spratt' and I wonder what an old lady like me might do to help. Was I right?"

"Avis, how did you . . . ? I mean, yes, you're right." Jane had to laugh. Trust Avis to skip all the drama and arrive at the same solution she and her friends had. The others stared, wide-eyed, dying to know what Avis was saying. "I'm going to Rocky Mountain Wildlife Hospital in Alberta," Jane continued, "to pick up enough vaccine to last us the summer."

"You're taking your sidekicks with you, I should hope!"

"Wouldn't leave home without 'em," she replied, grinning at her bewildered friends.

"Well then, it's a sound plan, missy. How can I help?" The line went silent as Avis waited for her answer.

"You would be a magical faerie, Avis, if you could assist us with a little matter of gas money . . ." She squeezed her eyes shut, knowing she was asking too much, and missing the sight of Amy, Flory, and Evie staring at her, openmouthed.

"Chump change!" was the astonishing reply. "Is that it?"

"Um, yeah. Yeah, Avis, that's it." Jane could hardly believe her ears. "Could you . . . meet me at my house in, oh, twenty minutes? Do you remember the way?"

They said their goodbyes, and Jane gently replaced

the receiver. Slowly, she looked up at her friends, the logistics of the next few hours already formulating themselves in her mind. "Evie, Ame, Flor, we leave here in my car via the back road and I loop around to the far side of the lake to drop Evie at her car. Then to my place to meet Avis, who is apparently bringing cash." She grinned now, giddy with the thrill of everything falling into place. "You've got your bags?" Amy and Flory lifted them into the air once again. Hers was in the car. They were ready to go.

Jane caught Amy glancing down at the trap door and knew she was thinking of Buster. "Ame," she said softly, "we'll be back by Monday. He'll be okay." Amy swallowed and nodded. "Cultus tonight, that gets us out of town unseen. Overnight at the MacGillivray cabin. We leave for Crowsnest Pass in the morning."

They traveled the underground passage to say their goodbyes to Mr. and Mrs. Mac, returned to blow out the candles one by one, and left under cover of darkness.

24

NO WORD FOR GOODBYE

JANE LEFT AMY AND FLORY at the MacGillivray cabin unrolling sleeping bags onto bunk beds and laying out breakfast things for morning and took the long trail up the western shore of Cultus Lake to Mountainview Country Club. The night was dark, darker than it ever got in the city, with no streetlights to outshine the stars, and she could just make out the lake, spilled ink at the bottom of a silk sky, still as a painting.

The security guard stopped her at the gate, and she fumbled for the right phrase, the secret password that would get her inside. In the end, she simply held up the flowers she'd brought and said, "For Audrey." He nodded and let her pass.

There were flowers on the lawn and on the stairs and in front of the door, lavish arrangements, simple bouquets, and hand-picked bunches of buttercups and clover tied with string. *Her grandchildren*, Jane thought. She climbed the stairs and laid her bundle with the others—pink and yellow roses from her mom's garden and cedar boughs from the trees near Elfin. Closing her eyes for a moment, she strove to recall all that Audrey had told her about crow medicine. *You're gonna live it,* she'd said. *Soon, I think.* Jane took a deep breath and let it out slowly. *No kidding, Audrey. Now if you could just stick close by a little longer . . . I don't think this is over quite yet.*

Rising at last, she turned to descend the stairs and found herself face to face with Jake Harbinsale. She let out a terrified yelp that brought the security guard running, flashlight beam panning across the length of Audrey's trailer. "Everything okay here, miss?" he called out. Jane stared into Jake's eyes and he returned her gaze. She was surprised and startled—so was he—but she wasn't afraid.

"Y-yes, thank you, sir!" she answered. The light receded, leaving them alone.

"Hi," he said finally, still holding her gaze.

"Hi," Jane responded softly. Chit chat was not her strong suit at the best of times, and it failed her utterly now.

Jake turned and sat down on the stairs, then held up a hand, inviting her to do the same. She took it, and settled next to him, keeping a little space between them. For a time, neither spoke. They gazed out at the lake, each seeing their own version of it.

"Here for the weekend?" he asked casually, still staring at the lake.

"No, I'm . . . Amy and Flory and I are . . . well, actually it's kind of a long story," she finished lamely.

"I've got time if you do," he said. And in a rush she remembered how he'd *always* had time for her, time to listen, time to talk over new ideas, time to help with whatever she was doing. It had been Jake who heard every detail of her campaign against SeaKing, and it had been Jake who helped her keep fighting when she was ready to give up.

She began at the beginning and left nothing out. He was silent until she finished, and then he uttered a low whistle. "Gee, Janey, first oil spills, now deadly viruses . . . can't you just go to the mall like normal girls?"

She turned sharply to check his expression and found him staring at her the way he used to, his eyes shining and his face soft the way he always looked back when . . . But that was then. And a lot had happened since, starting with his breakup with her by email. And then the silence . . .

"And you?" Her voice caught, and she cleared her throat. "Here for the weekend?"

"Well, no, not exactly," he hedged. "I've actually been here since Christmas—me and Bobby both." He paused. "Boo!"

She stared at him, her eyes wide. "*You're* the ghosts at the Harbinsale cabin? You and Bobby?" And then she laughed, hard, tears running down her face til she didn't know whether she laughed or cried. "Well, you "sure had everybody fooled!"

"Everybody except Audrey," he said, finally laying his own bunch of wildflowers down on the stoop. "I don't know how she figured us out, but she kept me from having to rob old Mr. Logan blind by bringing us food every day and leaving it by the back door. Every single day." He shook his head. "I used to laugh at her and call her awful names when I was Bobby's age. What a jerk I am."

Jane nodded and he laughed, a short, harsh sound. "No!" she said, suddenly realizing what he must have thought. "I meant we all were. None of us bothered to get to know her til . . . til it was almost too late."

"I *was* a jerk, Jane," he said fiercely, startling her. "I don't expect you to forgive me, or even understand, but I'm sorry. I felt awful. I didn't want to do it . . . what I did to you. But I couldn't . . . I was a coward." He put his face in his hands. "I couldn't stand up to him. Still can't." An involuntary shudder ran through him, and without thinking, Jane reached over and laid a soft hand on his back.

"Who, Jake?" she asked. "Who can't you stand up to?"

"My dad," he whispered through his hands. "Councilor Randall Harbinsale the Almighty, General Manager of Cedar's Ridge Golf & Country Club, man about town, head of the household, lord of all he surveys. He actually calls himself that as he drinks his orange juice in the mornings, standing at the kitchen door looking out over the backyard. My dad."

Jane nodded, understanding at least a little. She'd met Rand Harbinsale twice, and with his overbearing presence and mercurial shifts in mood, that was two times too many. "And so you left?" she pressed.

"I couldn't take the noise any more, Jane," he said. "The yelling over the phone at employees and suppliers, the sudden rages over a scuffed shoe or a lost tie, his face purple and the veins in his neck bulging whenever he lit into my mom or my little brother."

"And you," she added softly.

He nodded. "And me." He looked at her then. "You stood up to him, though, Janey. It drove him crazy! It was wonderful!" He gave her a wobbly smile.

"How do you mean?" she asked. "I ran crying from a Harbinsale family barbecue last fall, as I recall."

"The whole SeaKing thing!" he answered, as though it were obvious. "That mattered to him a lot for some reason. The owner was a friend of his, I think. And when the company folded, he was a dragon! It was awful around the house for weeks. It's what convinced me to leave, finally. But I was glad, Jane, glad that you won, glad that company had to pay to save those oiled animals."

She shook her head slowly, overwhelmed by what he was telling her. "But don't you see, Jake? I couldn't have done any of that without you. And you've stood up to him now—in the only way that was safe—by getting Bobby and yourself out of that situation." A sudden thought struck her: he'd actually tried to spare her a messy breakup, the "noise" of a confrontation, the thing he feared the most. He just hadn't realized that his silence, the sound she was all too familiar with in her own home, was what *she* feared the most.

Impulsively, she brought a hand to her throat and pulled the delicate silver chain out from under her sweater. The tiny feather pendant gleamed like a star in her hand. Jake caught his breath. "You still wear it? I thought you'd have ripped it off and flung it in the trash."

She laughed. "I did. But eventually I retrieved it and fixed it." She looked at him, knowing that even if she never again felt the way she had last fall, she'd always care about this boy. "You gave me a gift. Nothing changes that."

She tucked the pendant back inside her sweater, and as she did so caught a glimpse of her watch: almost midnight! "Jake, I've got to go!"

He nodded. "Me, too. Bobby's all alone in the cabin, and we've got to figure out where to go next. She left us some money with the last bag of groceries," he said, tapping his hand gently on the stair. "She must have known she was . . . I'm thinking maybe a bus trip, the Interior somewhere, we'll do a little camping." He saw the look on Jane's face. "We'll be okay, Janey. I've got relatives up there, and if things get that bad, we can always come back."

"Do you . . . want me to tell your family where you are?" Her mind flashed to the memory of Rand Harbinsale talking to Police Chief Emery in her dad's restaurant all those weeks ago. It had been Jake and Bobby they'd been talking about, she realized now. And Rand hadn't seemed to care all that much whether the Chief found his sons.

Jake shook his head emphatically, then paused. "I'd like my mom to know," he said softly, "if I didn't think my dad would . . . force it out of her." He looked up at Jane, as close to tears as she'd ever seen him. "Maybe, if you can find a way, just let her know we're okay." Jane promised she would.

He stood and held out his hand. She took it, and together they walked to the gates, where the path divided, and then they went their separate ways.

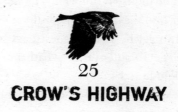

25

CROW'S HIGHWAY

FLORY DELAYED THEIR DEPARTURE SLIGHTLY when she pulled a clipboard out of her knapsack and announced that she would be taking inventory. Jane was rushing between the MacGillivray cabin and the car, loading their bags into the trunk, coolers of food and drink into the back seat, and maps and guide-books into the glove compartment. Amy sat slumped on a tree stump just outside the front door, disheveled curls hanging over her face, a raw strawberry pop tart gripped tightly in her hand. It was 3:40 a.m. Amy was not a morning person.

"Inventory . . . of what?" she growled from under her mane. "For what? Why?" She bit off a chunk of pop tart and chewed slowly.

"Insurance purposes!" Flory chirped, checking things off on her clipboard as Jane scooted by. "If someone should break into our vehicle and rob us, I will have a complete record of our personal possessions for the insurance company!"

"When exactly will this 'someone' have time to rob

us, Flory?" Jane inquired innocently as she stuffed their sleeping bags into the trunk. "According to the schedule you devised to get us to Crowsnest Pass before nightfall, we *might* get to pull over for a bathroom break *once* during daylight hours."

"Besides, they'd probably steal your inventory list, too," Amy muttered grumpily. "Ever think of that?"

Flory looked over at her sharply, clearly considering the idea for the first time, then slumped her shoulders in defeat and slipped her clipboard back into her bag. Sensing her disappointment, Amy pulled a small stack of CDs from her knapsack. "As long as we've got tunes and food, we've got everything we need, Flor."

Flory crouched by her own bag and lifted CDs out of the pocket, reading the names of the albums aloud. Jane waited til she'd finished, darkness hiding the sheepish look on her face, then said, "Uh, I hate to have to remind you of this at this exact moment in time, but my seventeen-year-old car only plays . . . cassettes."

Amy let out a wild groan and dropped her head to her knees. "Leave me here! Just leave me behind!"

"Well, let's see what you've got," Flory said optimistically. She reached into the glove compartment and emerged holding a single cassette. "Is this . . . is this all you brought, Jane? *Birdcalls of Southwestern British Columbia*? Oh my goodness, Amy, stop moaning like that or you'll wake the neighbors!"

"I thought I might . . . study," Jane confessed.

Bits of masticated pop tart flew from Amy's lips as she spoke from beneath her hair. "You have *got* . . . to be kidding me. We are *not* . . . listening to *that* : . . from here to *Alberta!*"

"Well then I guess you'll just have to sing!" Jane retorted as she slammed the trunk lid closed.

"Oooh, fun!" Flory clapped her hands gleefully as they got into the car. "Okay, everybody ready? Jane, you're the driver, obviously. I'll be the navigator and tour guide, since I've researched our route. And Amy, you'll . . . you can be . . . Amy, what are you?"

Amy stared at her balefully from her slouched position in the back seat. "I, Flory, am the dangerously cranky, sleep-deprived, and grossly undernourished ballast you brought along to weigh down the back end of the car." She glared at Jane. "I am also apparently your entertainment. And for that, you will both be very sorry."

Despite the delay, they pulled away from Cultus Lake just before dawn, before any light touched the far shore of the lake, before the crows awoke, before any birdsong broke the stillness of the new day. They stopped at a drive-thru in Chilliwack for hot cocoa, then joined the few other cars on the highway heading east.

They drove in silence for a while, Flory poring over the map, Amy dozing in the back, and as Jane caught sight of first light on the horizon ahead of her, she felt a tremor of nervous excitement in the pit of her stomach.

She could almost imagine they were embarking on a long summer holiday together, a thrilling cross-country adventure that would take them to mountain vistas and pristine parklands, past ancient glacial lakes and torrential rivers, and within view of ancient forest and rare wildlife. Almost. They *would* see all those sights, but at high speed, on fast forward, racing against time to retrieve the West Nile Virus vaccine from Rocky Mountain Wildlife Hospital and deliver it to the UWRC by Monday night. Three days. They had three days. And over 1,300 miles to travel.

At Hope, they pulled over for breakfast and to check the map. The first leg would take them on a high and winding journey across the crest of the Cascade Mountains and then down into the valley for a pit-stop in Princeton. The highway branched at Hope: the TransCanada led north toward Boston Bar; the Coquihalla northeast to Merritt; and the Number 3 east and south toward Manning Park and onward to their final destination. "There's your junction, Jane. Turn right here," Flory navigated from the passenger seat. "Crew, welcome to Highway 3, otherwise known as the Crowsnest Highway!"

"Crew you," Amy muttered from the back seat.

"Come again, Ame?" Flory challenged.

"I said," Amy spoke up, glancing back out the rear window, "we are now officially beyond Hope."

"Speak for yourself," Flory sniffed.

"Go back to sleep, Ame," Jane suggested, rolling her eyes. If the two of them sparred like this the whole way there, she'd be a wreck by nightfall. To her relief, she soon heard snoring from the back seat and checked her rearview mirror to find Amy blissfully unconscious, eyelids twitching, mouth open, head propped against a giant stuffed pink dog. Poor Ame. She had bravely refrained from mentioning Buster since last night, but Jane knew she was terribly worried about him. She felt a sharp pang of guilt as she thought of Sweet Pea and Minnie at home alone, with nothing but their overflowing food bowls and water fountains for company. *Well fed but starved for affection,* she thought miserably. *Or is that just me?* Well, only two more sleeps. At least at night they'd have her mom and dad to snuggle with.

She scanned the billboards as they flew by, beckoning her to all the exciting tourist attractions she wouldn't have time to see: Manning Park Lodge, the Cathedral Park campgrounds, the waterslides in . . . She laughed out loud, startling Flory. "Check it out, Flor," she said, pointing to the last billboard. It was the kind with the slats that rotated, and its mechanism had stalled, juxtaposing a very scantily clad male underwear model next to "The Scream Machine" triple loop waterslide. "Wish we had waterslides like that at home!" Flory giggled, craning her neck for a last look as they passed.

The highway soon started to climb, and they drove by a series of small lakes that fed into the Sumallo River.

"Hey Flor, those are Harlequin Ducks!" Jane exclaimed, thrilled to see the ornately feathered waterbirds in the wild. The only other time she'd seen Harlequins was in care at the wildlife center, after a canola spill in Burrard Inlet had coated them with oil.

"Home to the Spotted Owl," Flory said, pointing to a stand of giant, old-growth trees. "One of the rarest birds in Canada, possibly only twenty-three of them left. And twenty-two other species that share their forests are endangered as well." She sighed.

Flory spotted mountain goats on the far shore of the river and had Jane pull over so she could snap a picture. Back on the highway, she turned to Jane: "Smile!" and caught her friend at the wheel, long dark hair blowing about her shoulders, cedars, hemlocks, and Douglas firs blurring by in the background. She leaned into the back seat and composed "Sleeping Girl With Dog," then flipped the camera around and grinned into the lens. "Nostril shot," she giggled.

They passed through Manning Park and the highway began to climb again, twisting and turning around tight corners that had Jane gearing up and down and then up again just to keep her little car steady on the incline. At a barren break in the forest, which Flory said had been caused by a fire back in 1945, they felt as if they crossed an invisible line. The last of the early-morning clouds disappeared and the sky stretched blue and endless before them. "We're leaving the coastal forests behind,"

Flory explained, checking her notes, "and heading up into the subalpine. We'll follow the Similkameen River for the next hundred and twenty miles."

Jane and Flory took turns spying animals, Flory easily winning the game since Jane's attention was focused on keeping the car on the right side of the highway. Hot as it was already, and hot as it would get in her air-conditionless old sedan, she was glad of the dry conditions and the clear skies. And she was glad they'd left early enough that she would not have to navigate these twists and turns in the dark.

Amy woke as they rolled to a stop at a gas station in Princeton. Stepping out of the car, she yawned and stretched and within minutes was as perky as Flory had been at the start of the trip. "Woohoo!" she yelled up to the hills. "We're road trippin'! Let's do it!"

"We've been 'doing it' for several hours already, actually," Flory said, lips pursed. She was starting to feel the effects of their 3:00 a.m. rising time and was due for a little nap herself.

"Not with Amy Airlie MacGillivray, you haven't!" the voluble little redhead shouted, attracting the attention of the gas station attendants and a carload of university-aged boys. A few of them looked as though they'd be happy to join her party.

The girls took turns using the washroom, and Jane topped up the gas tank, thanking Avis again silently for her gift. After a quick snack and cold drinks from the cooler, they were back on the road.

"The Princeton-to-Osoyoos leg," Flory recited from her notes. "We will continue to follow the Similkameen River, and our route will take us by Nickel Plate Mountain and through Richter Pass, one of the nine passes we'll traverse today, and into the Okanagan Valley, where about a third of British Columbia's rare or endangered plants and animals make their home." Flory modulated her voice like a professional tour guide, sending Jane into fits of laughter. "Crew, please keep your eyes peeled for mountain goats and bighorn sheep, the tiny Mormon metalmark butterfly, long-billed curlews, bobolinks, and sage thrashers. Look as hard as you like, though, for white-tailed jackrabbits; the last time they were seen here was 1981."

Amy insisted Jane play *Birdcalls of Southwestern British Columbia* at full volume with the windows down. "We have very limited time to see wildlife, people," she said. "If we can't pull over and go to them, we'll just bring them to us!" Jane refrained from mentioning that they were now heading into south*eastern* British Columbia and therefore unlikely to have much success with the cassette. In any case, Amy was a talented mimic. Her promise to keep them entertained was not going unfulfilled.

"Swainson's Thrush," she said in an officious voice, striking the perfect note of academic superiority. And then: "Fuit, fuit, fuit, *fuit? What?*" She cleared her throat between birds. "Yellow Warbler: Sweet, sweet, sweet *shredded wheat!* Hey, peaches!"

"MacGillivray's Warbler?" Jane guessed, grinning.

"Seriously, Jane, we do break for peaches, don't we?" Amy implored.

Jane pulled the car over at one of the roadside stands that lined the highway as they approached Keremeos. Cherries, strawberries, and huckleberries, fragrant and warm under the late morning sun. "Lunchtime it is," she said, popping the trunk. She withdrew one of the sleeping bags and then collected the coolers from the back seat while Amy and Flory bargained for boxes of ripe Okanagan fruit. They found a quiet spot in one of the fields behind the stands, pulled sandwiches and cold drinks from the coolers, and spread open the sleeping bag for a feast.

After they'd eaten, Amy threw herself to the ground and announced, "I am so ready for a nap!"

"You just woke up!" Flory complained.

"Nap in the car," Jane sighed, "right after you help me clean all this stuff up. "And didn't we have some deal about singing?"

After a short stop in Osoyoos, they began to climb again, the little car struggling valiantly in the midday heat. They stopped at Haynes Point to stretch and to take in the triad of mountains on the western horizon: Mount Chopaka, Snowy Mountain, and Mount Kobau. "It's us!" Flory called, delighted, and asked another traveler to snap a photo of the three of them with the peaks in the background.

Back in the car twenty minutes later, they left the forest behind and started once again to descend. In the next valley, they found themselves on level ground for the first time since Princeton. Jane could practically feel her old car sigh with relief. But before long, they were climbing again.

Amy challenged Flory to a belching contest, which she won by default because Flory refused to participate. "Ugh!" Flory said as Amy started performing "99 Bottles of Beer on the Wall" without once using her vocal chords. Unbuckling her seatbelt, Flory crouched on her seat and stuck her head through the sunroof to breathe clean air.

"Sit down!" Jane yelled. "Flory, get back in here! Amy, stop that! Real singing only!"

"Gosh, Jane," Amy gushed, "you sound just like my mom. Ever think about having kids of your own? Okay, okay . . . Ninety-eight bottles of beer on the wall, ninety-eight bottles of beeeeeer," she sang, "if one of those bottles should happen to fall, there'd be ninety-seven bottles of beer on the wall. Ninety-seven . . ."

"A *real* song," Jane said through clenched teeth.

A noisy pair of crows flew from a copse of strange-looking trees on the slopes, the first crows they'd noticed or heard that day. "What are those trees, Flor, did your book say?"

"Trembling aspens," Flory replied, checking her notes. "A species of tree that rises up after a fire or other catastrophe. There was a smelter here that handled copper, silver, and gold ore from 1901 to 1918, and spewed enough sulfur dioxide to kill every tree for three miles around. As you can see, the forest still hasn't recovered."

And so of course the crow is here, Jane thought, recalling Audrey's words. *She has not the sing-song voice of other birds, and she tells not the sweet tales they tell. Her voice is harsh, and her stories are often so, as well.*

Amy started to sing the Beatles' "Blackbird," her voice low and quiet, barely audible over the hum of the car's engine. Jane and Flory listened, pressed into silence by the weight of the forest's past. *Take these broken wings and learn to fly.*

They climbed to Eholt Summit, finding themselves surrounded by western larch, white birch, Englemann spruce and soon, red cedar. Healthy forest. At Cascade, the highway turned north to Christina Lake, and there they stopped to dip their feet in the warm creek and watch the river jewelwing damselflies play over the water.

"Home stretch," Jane told them, checking her watch as they got back into the car. They were behind schedule and she wished, not for the first time, that they could just lift off like birds and fly, leaving all the turns and switchbacks of the highway behind. Onward to Castlegar, ascending again up the McRae Creek valley into subalpine forest, then a perilous descent to the Columbia River. At Castlegar, Amy pointed at the young trees on the hillsides: "Why no big trees here, Flor? Another fire?"

Flory shook her head. "Another smelter. Lead-zinc, in Trail, 1900 to 1940. Sulfur dioxide again." They stared out the window at the scar, gently bandaged in blue elderberry, lodgepole pine, white birch, mountain alder.

The highway descended again before turning east and upward to Kootenay Pass and into the Selkirk Mountains. "A whole gaggle of males? That's kind of weird, isn't it?" Amy asked, pointing out a herd of antlered caribou foraging for grasses and sedges in the meadow beside them.

"They're both," Flory answered, checking her notes.

"*Hermaphrodites?*" Amy exclaimed, incredulous. "I had no idea there were mammals that could . . ."

"No, idiot!" Flory squealed, laughing. "Both the males and the females have antlers—the only Canadian deer where that's the case. We're actually lucky to spot them. That's the only herd in this part of the province, and they're considered threatened."

"Geez, Flor, do you have any *good* news in that folder of yours?" Amy grimaced, staring out the window. "It's been all fires and smelters and clear cuts and animals on the brink of extinction since we left this morning." *This is Crow's highway,* Jane thought, listening to her friends' exchange. *Could that be part of Crow's message?*

"Coming up," Flory answered cryptically, then fell silent as the car chugged its way up and through Kootenay Pass, one of the highest in the province at 5,800 feet. Eking their way past the summit and a beautiful alpine lake, they all shared the car's relief as the highway began to descend yet again.

Flory picked up her folder once more. "Ladies and gentlemen . . ."

Amy snorted. "I wish!" Amy had called the boys at the last minute and invited them along on the trip, but both Ben and Mark had had to work this weekend. Flory had been philosophical about it, but Amy resented having to leave both her boyfriend *and* her dog behind.

"Ladies and Amy," Flory resumed, "welcome to the Creston Valley Wildlife Management Area, 7,000 hectares of marshland and one of the most important migration and breeding sites for water birds in the BC Interior. Tundra swans as well as thousands of ducks and coots pass through here each year, and the Valley is also nationally recognized for its breeding colonies of Forster's and Black Terns, Western, Eared, and Red-necked Grebes, and American Bitterns." She paused, casting a wary glance over her shoulder. "The northern leopard frog, once common throughout the Kootenays and south Okanagan, may now be found only in the Creston Valley marshes." She cleared her throat, hearing a rumbling in the back seat and unsure as to whether she should continue. "Uh, there are, um, you will also see Ospreys nesting here, although their numbers in North America fell dramatically in the second half of the twentieth century due to . . . pesticide poisoning."

"*Stop!*" Amy cried. "No more, Flory! I can't take the bad news, okay? Call me an eco-wimp, I don't care. Just . . . no more dying animals." To Flory's horror, Amy started to cry.

She looked quickly to Jane, who mouthed the word "Buster." It took her a moment to make the connection, and when she did, she felt terrible. "Oh, Ame, I'm so sorry! I didn't think . . . Amy, Buster is *not* going to die. He's not. He's getting the best possible care, and . . ."

"You don't know that, Flory," Amy said, wiping her face roughly. "Animals die all the time. You've been saying so yourself, all day long. And the wild ones . . . nobody's with them when it happens. Nobody sees it, nobody cares. Maybe that's why we all let it go on and on, this species gone, that species gone . . . forever!" She started to cry again. "But Buster . . . I always imagined I'd be there, you know? And now . . . now maybe I won't."

They drove for a time in near silence, Amy sniffling quietly in the back seat, Flory miserable in the front. Jane kept her eyes on the road signs, trying to get an idea of how far they had yet to go. She spotted a sign for Cranbrook, but if there'd been one for Crowsnest Pass, she'd missed it. Finally, Jane couldn't stand it any longer. She needed her navigator. She needed her friends. "Ninety-six bottles of beer on the wall," she started, "ninety-six bottles of beer, if one of those bottles should happen to fall, there'd be ninety-five bottles of beer on the wall."

"Not bad," Amy sniffed, "but you need to draw out that second 'beeeeer.' Like that. Take it from 'Ninety-five.'" Jane started singing again and Amy joined her, drawing out "beeeeeeeer" to ridiculous lengths that finally got Flory laughing.

The three of them made it all the way to fifty-two bottles before Jane said, "Flor, where on planet Earth are we, exactly?"

"Rocky Mountain Trench," Flory answered without pause, as though she'd been keeping up her commentary inside her head, "the greatest of all geological structures in British Columbia." In the warm light of the setting sun, the valley was indeed impressive, and when Flory told them that it stretched all the way from the Yukon down to northern Montana, they stared around them in wonder.

"I guess we're actually pretty lucky to see all this," Amy admitted, the sheer age and scope of the Trench forcing her to look with new eyes. "To see any of it— before it's gone."

Flory read off the key landmarks as they rolled up and down hills and began to climb once again. Coming to the Elk River, flowing south to Montana, Flory said,

"We go the other way," and she pointed upward, "into the Rocky Mountains." And suddenly, there they were.

Surrounded at home by Vancouver's local peaks, the girls were used to the sight of mountains at close range. But nothing could have prepared them for the Rockies. Towering, untamed, sky-scraping crags of pre-historic rock and ice, these mountains were wild things, forces of nature, alive and seeming to rise and climb still, forced upward by the same unseen thrust of sub-terranean energy that earthquakes and volcanoes were made of.

"We're going *there?*" Jane squeaked, utterly awed. "My little car has to go all the way up *there?*"

"Onward!" Flory commanded. And on they went. And up. The little car chugged and Jane geared down, hugging the right side of the highway and letting faster cars pass them by. They entered a tunnel and Amy hollered at them to lift their feet off the floor and put their hands on the roof and scream the whole way through for good luck. Jane kept her hands and feet on the gear shift and the pedals, but obligingly screamed her throat raw. They emerged on the eastern slope of the Lizard Range, laughing hysterically.

"These mountains are upside down," Flory said off-handedly as she re-opened her folder in what was left of the day's light.

"Um, Flor?" Amy was still wheezing. "You sure you didn't just accidentally flip your folder upside down while we were in the tunnel?"

"Whatever geological catastrophe pushed the Rocky Mountains up out of the earth flipped the Lizards at the same time," Flory answered, undeterred. "The rock at their peaks is a hundred and ten million years older than the rock at their bases . . . give or take."

"Hey, Jane," Amy said, leaning into the front seat, "next time some other driver does something really dumb, flip 'em the lizard!" They laughed at that until an overhead sign turned their laughter into cheering: You Are Entering the Municipality of Crowsnest Pass.

The light in the sky was fading quickly, and as the streetlights in the little town flickered on, they used them to read the signs. Just past a friendly looking diner, they spotted the one they were looking for: Rocky Mountain Wildlife Hospital, 2 Miles, Next Exit. Jane turned off the main street and they found themselves on a rough, narrow, unlit road leading into the brush.

"We're here, we're here, we're here!" Flory squealed, bouncing in her seat as the car bumped its way through potholes and over unseen obstacles in the road. At that moment, Jane heard an alarming hiss in the front end and simultaneously saw her dashboard light up like a slot machine hitting the jackpot. There was a terrible rattle, and then billowing clouds of steam emerged from the front of the car, completely obscuring their view. Jane just had time to pull the car over to the side of the road before it gave one last shudder and died.

26

A NIGHT IN THE CROW'S NEST

N O ONE SPOKE as they unloaded their packs and sleeping bags from the trunk of the car and set off on foot along the dark dirt road. Jane walked in the middle, Amy on her left, Flory on her right, each girl carrying a flashlight and glad of the stars, each one lost in thoughts about time, distance, the task ahead of them, the journey home.

Jane's car was clearly out of commission, but for how long? Tomorrow was Sunday on a long weekend. Would there be anyone in this little town willing to do the necessary repairs? And even if there were, how would they pay for them? The girls had planned to spend Sunday morning in Crowsnest Pass to give Jane a chance to rest before commencing the grueling journey back over the Rockies and across the province to Cedar's Ridge. Flory had set their departure time for 1:00 p.m., and they had reserved a campsite in Osoyoos for Sunday night, with the intention of completing the last half of the trip by mid-afternoon Monday. It was do-able, though tight. But now?

Jane knew Amy was thinking of Buster, of just how far away she was from him, and now, how stuck. She wished suddenly that she'd left Amy back in Cedar's Ridge, close by in case Buster . . . If something did happen, she couldn't imagine how she'd live with herself. Just as suddenly, she heard Avis's voice in her head, sharp and strident as if her imperious old friend were right there with her: *No use wishing away reality, missy. Play the hand you've been dealt!*

Jane thought then of all the animals currently in care at the UWRC and of the Center's decision to accept corvids again come Tuesday morning. If the birds were carrying West Nile Virus, as experts predicted they would be this summer, they would put every animal in the hospital in grave danger. She was here in Alberta with Amy and Flory to pick up a controversial vaccine that had the potential to minimize that danger and save lives. They'd made it too far to fail now because of a broken-down car. Somehow, they had to get back to Cedar's Ridge with the medicine before Tuesday. The question was, how?

Lights twinkled through the trees in the distance, and Jane picked up her pace. Those weren't stars. That was the Rocky Mountain Wildlife Hospital. And somebody was still up, awaiting their arrival.

Shelley Eggars greeted them like prodigal daughters and had them wrapped in blankets by the fireplace, mugs of hot tea in their hands and fresh-baked scones laid out on the low pine coffee table before they'd barely said hello. Jane thought she'd never felt so warm, nor tasted food so good.

"Now, tell me all about your trip!" Shelley said, plumping herself down on the couch and then instantly jumping back up again. "No, wait, let me email Evie first and let her know you've made it safe and sound." She bustled away into a little alcove at the back of the tiny cabin. "I've put mattresses up in the loft for tonight. I'll sleep down here on the couch. Don't worry, it happens all the time. I'm practically an extra hotel here in the Crow."

As Jane watched her go, pure energy clothed in a navy-blue hoody and sweats, messy blond ponytail poking out from under an old ball cap, she thought, *She's just like Evie. Thinner, taller, older maybe, fast-moving to Evie's slower, deliberate ways. But here she is living in a log cabin in the middle of nowhere, with a wild animal hospital out back. This is home. Nothing matters more than the animals.* She felt a surge of confidence. If anybody could help them do what they came here to do, Shelley Eggars could.

"Shelley, is that . . . are those . . . ?" Jane was pointing to a stack of cardboard cartons piled beside the stairs leading up to the loft.

"Enough vaccine to last you all the way through mosquito season," Shelley confirmed, rejoining them by the fire. "It arrived here yesterday from Manitoba.

They shipped as soon as Evie's payment went through." She shook her head as she munched on a hot buttered scone. "We're such a sleepy little town here, and West Nile's such old news for us, it's hard to imagine all the hoopla that's been raging out your way. If I hadn't seen the protests and signs and fights on TV, I wouldn't have believed it. So tell me, what's your itinerary for tomorrow? Are you up at the crack of dawn for an early departure?"

"Well," Jane said, glancing at the others, "as a matter of fact, we've hit a bit of a roadblock . . . so to speak." And together with Amy and Flory, she related the details of their journey east, ending with her car's sudden demise and their two-mile walk to Rocky Mountain.

"I see," Shelley said slowly as she cleared away the plate and mugs. "Well, well, well . . . it's almost midnight on the Saturday of a long weekend, and nothing opens in the Crow on a Sunday til at least eleven. The way I see it, you'd best get a good sleep now, and we'll rise and shine and tackle the problem tomorrow over a big brunch. You've done all you can do for one day." She started washing dishes, her back to the girls. "Bathroom's under the stairs, help yourself to anything you need, and I'll holler for you in the morning after I've fed the animals." She spread her own sleeping bag out on the couch as the girls headed upstairs to the loft.

Shelley was right. There was nothing more to be done tonight. Still, Jane couldn't help lying awake, tossing in the heat, staring up at the vaulted ceiling over the loft, and going over and over the problem in her mind. She could hear Amy downstairs in Shelley's office, typing what sounded like a very long, very urgent email to someone—maybe Ben, maybe Mike, who was at home with Buster. Minutes or hours later, she finally fell asleep, the sound of tapping on keys entering her dreams like rain.

27

LEAVE IT TO BEAVER

By 4:30 SUNDAY AFTERNOON, they were frantic. Jane had had the car towed to Biddley's Auto in town that morning, which had bitten a big chunk out of Avis's gas money. Shelley had offered to cover repair costs up to $500 and arranged for Jane to pay her back over the rest of the summer with money she made at her job. Arthur Biddley had promised to do his best to complete any mechanical work by mid-afternoon, but couldn't make any guarantees. And according to an email from Mike, Buster was back in the hospital.

One o'clock came and went. Then two o'clock. Then three o'clock. Jane called Biddley's: "Won't be long now," Arthur Biddley had said. But now it was 4:30. They had three and half, maybe four hours of real daylight left. They might make it to Creston, but they wouldn't get anywhere near Osoyoos, and Monday would be a harrowing race back to the city.

They were sitting around the kitchen table, anxious and silent, when the phone rang. Everyone jumped. "Go ahead, Jane," Shelley said, waving a hand at the phone.

"It's gotta be him."

"Urban Wild . . . er . . . Rocky Mountain Wildlife Hospital, Jane Ray speaking," she said. "Yes, hello Mr. Biddley! Oh . . . well, good news first, I guess." She glanced around the table, shrugging. "I'm sorry, did you say Wednesday? But remember I said . . . but can't you . . . wouldn't they . . . there's no way . . . ?" She saw Amy's face turn a sickly shade of white. "Sir, if that's the good news, what's the bad . . . ? *What?* A whole new eng . . . twenty-five hund . . . oh . . . oh my . . ." She turned her back on the three anxious faces. "I'll . . . how about I call you back when I decide what to do. You're open til five? All right, then. Thank . . . yes, sir, thanks very much, Mr. Biddley."

She hung up the phone and turned slowly back to face her friends, her hands clenched at her sides. Looking directly at Amy, whose eyes were glassy with unshed tears, she said, "Not only has he not finished repairing the car, he hasn't even started. It needs . . . it overheated. The gaskets are all blown. It's got to have a whole new engine, which he can't get til Wednesday. And it's going to cost twenty-five hundred dollars. More than my dad paid for the car in the first place." She paused. "I'm not . . . it's a write-off." She cleared her throat, and went on, clearly and quietly. "We'll take the Greyhound bus home tomorrow, and we'll take the vaccine with us. I'll pay for the tickets. Ame, I'll get you home."

"Jane," Shelley broke in softly, "it's a long weekend.

The buses will be packed. Let me call the station." She was off the phone in minutes, shaking her head. "Not a single seat, nothing til Tuesday morning. Would you like me to reserve three?"

"That won't be necessary, Shelley, but thanks anyway," Amy interrupted, her voice sounding high and strangely loud in the small cabin. "We'll hitchhike, starting tonight."

Jane, Shelley, and Flory all spoke at once. "Amy, that's crazy!" "That's illegal and dangerous. I can't let you do that." "Think, Amy—it could take you longer to get home instead of shorter—if you get there at all!"

"*I'm going!*" Amy shouted, the tears falling now. "You can sit here helpless with your precious vaccine for another day if you want, but I'm going home to my dog!" She tore across the room and bounded up the stairs to the loft, sobbing as she stuffed her things into her knapsack.

Jane stared down at her hands, defeated. *Where's Crow now?* she thought. *Hey, Audrey?* She could hear the old woman's voice in her head, mocking her. *Those who need her medicine will find her at crossroads, in the dark places, and at the gateway between living and dying. Those who seek her will always find her, and she will show them the way home.* She gazed over at the boxes of vaccine piled by the stairs, and listened to Amy's muffled sobs. *Thanks for nothing, Old Crone.*

"Open up, or I'll huff and I'll puff and I'll blow your

house down!" A thunderous pounding shook the cabin as a bellowing male voice called from outside.

"Ralphie!" Shelley cried and ran to the door. It swung open to reveal a bear in mountain man's clothing—a giant barrel of a man in a Macintosh and cap, denims and boots, dirt and engine oil under his fingernails and a weathered face split by a wide grin. He lifted Shelley off the floor and swung her around in a crushing hug.

"Hoo, boy, ain't you a sight for sore eyes, lady! Hyeh, hyeh!" He held her out from him, eyes alight with pleasure, then pulled her in close for a lengthy kiss.

She backed away from him at last, blushing and brushing imaginary lint from her sleeve. "Ralph, I've got company. I wasn't expecting you for another week!"

Ralph shared his grin with Jane and Flory, and doffed his cap, "How d'ye do, ladies! Hyeh, hyeh! Ralph Mailer, semi-retired bush pilot and the luckiest man in the world!" He grabbed Shelley and gave her another quick kiss. "What's for dinner?"

Shelley was already bustling about the kitchen, turning on burners and pulling ingredients from shelves and cupboards. Without waiting for answers, Ralph tossed his cap onto a chair and slung his Mac over the back, then sat himself down with the girls. "I was camping in just about the prettiest spot in the country, ladies. You ever get the chance to spend some time on Kootenay Lake, you jump at it! All by my lonesome, just me and the wild west, beautiful weather, another whole week to go, when these danged crows start waking me up in the morning and harassing me all the livelong day, giving me not one minute's peace from morning til night! Two days I stood it, and that was that. And besides," he winked at Shelley, "they got me thinking about my girl stuck here in the Crow with the animals and nobody to give her a break. And so I thought, Why not spend my second week with Shell? So here I am!" He slammed his enormous hands down on the kitchen table. "We're getting married come September, Shelley and I, did she tell you that? No? Well, it's true, and we're gonna honeymoon wherever the wind takes us. Be my second time, her first, and what a catch like her wants with a divorced old granddaddy like me I will never know, but life is a funny thing, girls. Now then! This looks like a party somebody just pulled the plug on. What's your story? And say," he narrowed his eyes and pointed at Jane, "haven't I seen you on TV?"

It was all the opening Jane needed. She poured out her tale to Ralph Mailer from beginning to end, Flory filling in the few details she missed, and when they finished, he sat back in his chair and folded his arms. "That the cargo there?" he asked, indicating the boxes of vaccine against the back wall. Jane nodded. "And there's just the two of you?"

"Er, three," Jane said, glancing toward the loft.

Ralph looked over at Shelley, who was staring back at him from the kitchen. "Are you at least going to stay for dinner?" she asked, suspending her preparations.

Jane looked back and forth between the two of them, barely breathing. Could he be thinking what she thought she was thinking? She couldn't ask, not for something so big. But if he were to offer . . .

"I pilot a 1952 DeHavilland Beaver floatplane, girls," Ralph said with evident pride, "an eight-seater with four seats removed for cargo, which leaves four for us. How would you like to fly home?"

Flory clamped her hands to her mouth to muffle her squeals. Jane closed her eyes, grinning, and offered up a silent thank you. Then she looked up to the loft: "Ame?"

A tuft of red curls appeared over the railing, and then two round, slightly puffy blue eyes: "Let me check my schedule."

Shelley made burgers and deep-fried onion rings with dill pickles and red-pepper mayonnaise on the side for dipping. "Ralphie's favorite," she smiled. Ralph had four. After dinner, they sat together around the coffee table poring over maps, and Ralph showed them the route they'd fly in the morning.

"You'll be home in time for lunch," he told them. "And I'll be back in time for dinner." He winked at Shelley and she blushed. He glanced at his watch, then stretched and yawned loudly. "Bedtime, ain't it?"

28

JANE LEARNS TO FLY

RALPH SHOUTED TO THEM to put their headsets on as he made one last inspection of the cockpit with the engine running and the propeller turning. And then they were taxiing across Crowsnest Lake, liquid runway visible only to their pilot, propeller tips howling as they approached the speed of sound. "We need maximum horsepower to clear the water," Ralph spoke into his microphone, pointing to a needle on the instrument panel that was inching toward the red line. "But this baby's so smooth, hyeh, hyeh, you won't even know we're in the air til you look down and see the treetops!"

They'd said their thanks and goodbyes to Shelley over a lumberjack's breakfast of bacon, eggs, sausages, and pancakes early that morning. The girls had stuffed themselves with flapjacks and strawberries. Ralph had polished off the rest. Shelley helped them load the cartons of vaccine into Ralph's pickup truck while Ralph filed their flight plan with Canadian Flight Service, and then they were off, Rocky Mountain Wildlife Hospital disappearing behind them at a bend in the road.

At Crowsnest Lake, they'd spotted the floatplane at once bobbing jauntily at the dock, her white body and crisp green trim sparkling in the morning sun. Despite the plane's age, Ralph explained that she'd been designed to operate in rugged bush country and in freezing weather, and her simple, solid construction had stood the test of time. Just over five thousand pounds of pure metal, four-hundred-and-fifty-horsepower Pratt & Whitney R-985 radial engine, high-lift wings extending straight out from the top of the body, prop at the nose and seaplane fins at the tail, all resting on EDO 4930 floats. Designed and built in Canada, the DeHavilland Beaver was considered by many to be the best bush plane ever made.

While Ralph completed his pre-flight inspection, they'd stowed the vaccine and their gear behind the seats with a little room to spare, then they strapped themselves in, Ralph in the pilot's seat and Jane to his right, Amy behind him and Flory behind Jane. And they were off.

Amphibian to avian, the Beaver brushed the surface of the mountain lake like wind over glass, and it was only by sensing a slight acceleration as the floats left the water that Jane guessed they were airborne.

The little plane climbed slowly, taking its time to leave the Nest, but before long they had a bird's-eye view of the journey they had taken just two days before.

Like ants they'd been, crawling through this vast, magnificent landscape, seeing it in pieces, fragments. Now they flew above it, seeing it whole.

Jane was struck by the vivid colors—the verdant limes and kellies and loden greens of the trees and forests, the crystalline blues and turquoises of the lakes and sky—and by the shapes and patterns that were imperceptible from the ground but as readable from the air as words on a page. She thought of how the very lines on the face of someone you loved were lovable, too. *I love this,* she realized, *now that I've known it from above and below, now that I've seen it like this.* She'd often wondered how birds made their lengthy migrations with little more than instinct to guide them. Looking down now, she understood that they must be intimately familiar with every feature of the Earth along their path, that they must love her, must find their way easily to the particular lines and shapes and colors they called home.

Almost as good a tour guide as Flory, Ralph delighted in pointing out quirky landmarks and telling horror stories about landslides and mining disasters. Jane looked left, then right, then left again in an attempt to follow his narrative, and before too long she found herself sickeningly nauseous. Trying to hide her discomfort, she faced forward and took slow, deep breaths, but to her embarrassment, the nausea grew worse.

Ralph soon noticed he'd lost a member of his audience. "Got the queasies?" he chuckled. She nodded and instantly regretted the movement. "Want to know the best instant cure for that?" She made a small "hmm" sound she hoped would pass for "yes." She didn't dare open her mouth. Out of the corner of her eye, she saw him loosen a bolt at the hub of the steering mechanism, and suddenly he was lifting the wheel over the center-line of the cockpit, setting it in front of her, and bolting it into place. "Take the wheel for a while—always works for me!"

Jane flew them the rest of the way home, following Ralph's instructions: Eyes on the horizon line, now; a little to the left; easy right, gently; nose up, higher, higher, Jane, the floats have to clear that mountaintop, too!; nose down, steady, that's a girl, you got 'er. After twenty minutes or so, nausea forgotten, cold sweat dried to salt on her face, she was able to loosen her grip on the wheel and relax her shoulders, and that's when it hit her: she was flying! Sure, she'd been in planes before, and maybe that's what this sensation was, but the strange thing was that the feeling wasn't foreign . . . it was familiar. Ralph kept control of the throttle—the power—but she had the rudders. Nose, wings, and tail were hers. She was flying.

If she'd thought the trip up to Crowsnest Pass had been a race, it was nothing compared to their return trip home. Despite the urgency of their mission, she was suddenly a little sorry it would be over so soon. Over the Rockies with a fond wave to the Lizard Range; across the

Rocky Mountain Trench and into the Purcells; grazing the serene greens of the Creston Valley; some careful navigation through the airspace over Castlegar airport; over the Monashee Mountains and Christina Lake into the Kettle Valley; a hello to their trio of peaks near Osoyoos; over the wilds of Cathedral Provincial Park and Manning, with an awe-inspiring look at the long-winding Similkameen. A few minutes later, her heart leapt. That was Cheam Peak, and Chilliwack River, and the outline of *that* lake was as familiar to her as the lines of her own face. Cultus.

They were slated to land in the busy inner harbor in downtown Vancouver, so it wouldn't be long before they'd have to begin their descent. Jane glanced left to check in with Ralph and indicate she was ready to pass the controls back to him. He was reaching to flip a switch on the control panel that read "Multicom." Turning to her, his face ashen and slick with sweat, he lifted a hand to his heart and then dropped it again, a dead weight. His breath gurgled in his throat and his eyelids fluttered. Then he slumped in his seat, unconscious.

29

EMERGENCY PROCEDURES

FOR A LONG MOMENT, THERE WAS SILENCE. No sound at all—no engine, no prop, not even the beating of her own heart as Jane stared at their pilot, uncomprehending. Then, as though she were bursting into air from deep under water, she came to in the cabin, to the sound of Flory screaming.

"Fly the plane! Jane, oh, holy mother help us, Jane, fly the plane!" Flory screamed from behind her.

"Charlie Foxtrot nine one five, we read. What is your destination?"

They were headed straight for a stand of cedars. The voice in her headset would have to wait. Crashing on three, two, and . . . Jane gripped the wheel and tilted it back hard, too hard, pulling them up in a sickening lift that caused the plane to shudder and jolt. *Breathe,* she told herself, tossing her head to fling the sweat from her eyes. *Breathe. You did this before. Do it again.* Gently, she pressed forward on the wheel and brought the nose down to even them out.

"Charlie Foxtrot nine one five, this is Vancouver

Terminal. Do you read? Acknowledge."

"Flory, look at me. Stop screaming." It was Amy, out of her seat, her hands on Flory's shoulders. "Look at me. I need you. Do you think you can help me?" Flory put a hand to her mouth and nodded. "Good. We're going to get Ralph out of the cockpit and onto the floor behind our seats, okay? Undo your seatbelt, then undo his, okay? Got it? All right, let's go."

"Charlie Foxtrot nine one five, this is Vancouver Terminal. We have you on radar. Are you requesting permission to land?"

"Mayday," Jane whispered, unable to find her voice. "Mm . . . mayday. Can you hear me? Please help." She could see the Fraser River below them, and the city of Abbotsford on their left. The plane seemed to be flying itself, with little nudges now and then from her. But it couldn't stay up here forever. She glanced wildly at the instrument panel, scanning for the fuel gauge. How much time did they have? In her peripheral vision, she watched Amy and Flory strain to manoeuver Ralph out of his seat and onto the floor—a mountain of dead weight that moved in agonizing slow motion. How much time did *he* have?

Amy pushed him sideways by the shoulders and Flory dragged him by his right arm until he tumbled awkwardly onto his side between the seats. Sweating heavily, the two girls stepped over him and met at his head, where together they reached under his arms and inched him along the floor to the back of the cabin.

"I've got him, Flory," Amy said. "Go navigate, okay? Get us down. We need an ambulance. Go. Flor, I said, *go!*"

"Charlie Foxtrot nine one five, is there a problem? We do not read. I say again, is there a problem?"

Flory slid into Ralph's seat and slipped on his headset. "You . . . you're doing great, Jane," she said, her voice shaking.

"Flory, somebody's trying to reach us, and I can't make them hear me," Jane said. "Please, please, can you help me figure it out?"

"Ralph, can you hear me?" Amy was kneeling beside Ralph, one hand on his forehead and the other on his chin. "Ralph, can you hear me?" she repeated.

"Charlie Foxtrot nine one five, where are you flying from and what is your intended destination? Please report to Vancouver Terminal *immediately.*"

Amy swept a finger through Ralph's mouth checking for obstructions and, finding none, pinched his nostrils closed, tilted his chin up and breathed into his mouth, watching for his chest to rise and fall. Yes. The airway was clear. But he still wasn't breathing on his own. Or moving. At all. Something blocking circulation. Begin chest compressions.

Flory looked over at Jane, studying her headset, then reached for her own and ran her fingers along the curved metal band that held the microphone in front of her mouth. There. She pressed the button in and spoke:

"Mayday, mayday. This is Ralph Mailer's plane. We have an emergency. Uh, over." She released the button.

Amy crouched over Ralph, her hands on his sternum. "And one, and two, and three, and four . . ." She pushed down on his chest with every one of her hundred and ten pounds, fifteen compressions, then bent to breathe for him again.

"Charlie Foxtrot nine one five, this is Vancouver Terminal." The voice was extremely calm. "Roger mayday. Who is flying Ralph Mailer's plane? And where is Ralph?"

"And nine, and ten, and eleven, and twelve . . ."

"Jane Ray is flying the plane, sir," Flory responded. "She is seventeen years old and does not know how to fly, but she is doing an excellent job so far." She smiled tremblingly over at Jane. "Ralph is unconscious and another member of our party is administering CPR, but we need paramedics. Over. *Now.* Over."

"This is Vancouver Terminal. Say again. We did not hear you correctly. Say again."

"And one, and two, and three, and four . . ."

Jane grabbed her headset and squeezed the microphone button. "This is Jane Ray. You heard correctly. The pilot is down and a teenager is flying the plane."

There was silence over the multicom, then static. And then: "Vancouver Terminal to Jane Ray. We have alerted all aircraft in local airspace to your situation. You have clearance to land in Vancouver harbor immediately. We will instruct your landing from the ground. Emergency crews will be on hand."

For all of us, Jane thought. Then she deliberately turned her mind from the terror that lay ahead. She couldn't think about landing, not yet. Scanning the horizon for familiar landmarks, she identified Langley on their left, Maple Ridge on their right, Surrey, Coquitlam, and New Westminster spreading out ahead of them. The downtown harbor was at least another fifteen minutes away. Ralph didn't have that kind of time.

"And five, and six, and seven, and eight . . ."

She glanced back at Amy and Ralph and then over to Flory, and shook her head. Flory understood at once. She spoke into the mic: "This is Flory Morales, navigator for Jane Ray, calling Vancouver Terminal. Request permission to land sooner. Like, now."

Silence, then static. "Verify position, Flory Morales."

She looked down. "We are directly over the border between New Westminster and Cedar's Ridge."

"And twelve, and thirteen, fourteen, fifteen . . ." Amy's continued efforts meant that Ralph still wasn't breathing on his own, still had no circulation. Might already be . . .

"Vancouver Terminal to Flory Morales. Alter course northeast into Cedar's Ridge. Permission granted to land immediately on Aerie Lake. Emergency crews are being dispatched now. Do you read?"

Jane shook her head in wonderment. Aerie Lake, site

of the Urban Wildlife Rescue Center. Hub of the storm, home to thousands of protestors for weeks, focus of the controversy that had sent them into the mountains in secret in the first place. Well, there would be no secret delivery of the vaccine today. All the world would hear them coming—and see them succeed, or fail . . . spectacularly. She turned to Flory and gave a slight nod before tilting the wheel slightly up and to the right, toward home.

"Flory Morales to Vancouver Terminal. We read. Approaching Aerie Lake for landing."

"And one, and two, and three, and four . . ."

Avis Morton was peeling apples in her kitchen and listening to the radio as she watched birds flit around the feeders she'd hung in her backyard. George always loved a juicy crumble for dessert, extra cinnamon. She wondered when she'd be able to return to her shift at the UWRC. This nonsense had gone on long enough. She missed the animals. The girls were due back today with the vaccine. Maybe that would ease the tension.

When the eleven o'clock news started, she reached out to shut it off. Nothing but doom and gloom, usually. "Our top story this morning: Will it be a 'crash course' in flying? A floatplane pilot has been incapacitated in mid-flight from southern Alberta and Cedar's Ridge teen Jane Ray is at the controls. There are two other passengers on board. With guidance from the ground, Ms. Ray will attempt to land the plan on Aerie Lake in Cedar's Ridge, and emergency crews have been dispatched to the scene. We'll follow that story live to its conclusion, so please, stay with us. For CKTS Radio in Vancouver, this is Linda Vir . . ."

Avis's hands flew to her heart. Missy? Flying a plane? For goodness' sake, she'd given her plenty of money for gas. After a moment's hesitation, she whirled, snatching her keys from the kitchen counter, and hurried to her car. She'd get to the UWRC this morning if she had to mow those protestors down herself.

Mike snuggled with Katrina on the den couch, ignoring the TV and listening with one ear for the phone. They had the house to themselves, which *never* happened. His parents were at Cultus for the long weekend, his sister had left town on a road trip, and his dog was in the hospital again. If the vet called with good news, he was going to take Katrina downtown to watch the fireworks. But every time Buster went into the hospital, it became less and less likely that he would make it out again. It was shaping up to be another night of his dubious cooking and waiting by the phone. He'd bought a few rockets and firecrackers just in case they ended up celebrating by themselves in the backyard, but he doubted Kat would be impressed.

"The young woman flying the plane has identified herself as Jane Ray, and the two other teenagers with her as Florencia Morales and Amy MacGillivray." Mike bolted upright on the couch and reached for the remote, cranking the volume. What the . . . Staring at the screen, he saw a small white floatplane with green trim, Cedar's Ridge below in the background. Judging by the sounds, it was being filmed by a helicopter flying alongside. Live. This was live.

Katrina sat up beside him, straightening her clothes. "And you call *me* a drama queen," she tried to joke, but her words fell flat.

"As if the challenge ahead of her weren't great enough, Toni, our camera crew on site at Aerie Lake informs me that protestors have headed out onto the lake in rowboats to try to prevent her landing," the reporter announced. The screen flashed a shot of Aerie Lake from the dock behind the wildlife center, where swarms of protestors had moved up from the road to surround the Care Center and line the lakeshore. Five or six boats were making their way toward the middle of the lake. "Whether they don't understand that the real pilot is in critical condition, or that an inexperienced teen is flying that plane, I cannot say. But the situation looks grim indeed. Back to you, Toni."

"Thanks, Ed. We'll continue to follow that story as . . ."

"Oh my god!" Katrina gasped, fully alert now. "She

must've gone for the vaccine! After all Evie's warnings! Is she crazy?"

"We gotta get down there," Mike exclaimed, leaping to his feet. "We've got to do something!" He tore into the basement, looking around wildly for something useful to take with him to the lake as he yanked on his sneakers. "You coming, Kat?" Or maybe do you want to stay here in case the vet calls? Kat?"

"Mike." She stood at the entrance to the basement, watching him search frantically for god-knows-what hand-held power tool he thought would help him land an airplane from the ground. "Come watch with me. There's nothing we can do." She reached out, grabbing his hand, and pulled him back into the den.

"What do you mean, there's nothing . . . Kat, it's my sister! It's . . . it's . . . oh, god." He sat heavily, his head in his hands, unable to look at the TV screen but unable to block out the newscaster's endless stream of words or the drone of the little plane.

"It's Jane Ray," Katrina finished his sentence, so quietly the newscast drowned out her words. Still holding his hand, she watched, and he listened, and the words went on, and on.

The drone of the floatplane's engine and the ominously low chop of the helicopter had brought the bulk of the protestors up the access road to the UWRC.

They had rightly guessed that the controversial WNV vaccine was going to be delivered by air and had made up their minds to prevent it if they could. Newscasts had also brought the animal rights protestors of previous weeks back to the lake, determined to stop the others from blocking the delivery of the vaccine. The ensuing commotion brought lakeside residents out onto their porches and docks, hands raised against the sun's glare as they gazed up at the flying machines and across the lake at the growing crowds. Aerie Lake was ringed with people, all looking up at the sky.

Jane circled the lake once more, shaking from the strain, sweating again, trying to keep the instructions straight. Of course, none of it would matter if those rowboats didn't clear the lake. She couldn't land on top of them, but she was running out of fuel. *And out of time.* Behind her, Amy counted, and breathed, tireless.

Flory talked through the procedure with her again as she circled, the repetitions calming her slightly. She'd had a helicopter on her tail for the past two or three minutes, and its presence in her peripheral vision wasn't helping her nerves. At first, she'd thought it was some kind of rescue crew, but then she'd spotted the camera. Unbelievable. They were going to film her landing. Or her crash landing. Didn't matter to them. In fact, a crash would make for better ratings.

Enough. Focus. Review. Repeat. She looked down. They were still there, a little flotilla in the middle of the lake, holding them hostage in the air. She was half way through her circle and directly over the dock behind the UWRC. It was so weighted down with screaming protestors that it was half submerged in the lake. Even if she got the plane down, how would they ever get Ralph out of here? No, not if. *When.* When, when, when.

She completed her clockwise circle at the far end of the lake, praying that when she turned the floatplane around, somehow the scene would have changed, that the lake would be clear, that she could land. As she banked right, angling the plane to face the dock, Jane spotted the swirling red and white lights of police cars and ambulances as they skidded to a stop at the head of the access road. She could just make out the low, nasal squawk of a voice through a bullhorn—*emergency, pilot down, teenager*—ragged quarks reminding her, bizarrely, of the calls of a crow. *Those who need her medicine will find her at the gateway between living and dying.*

And then all at once, the boaters on the lake scattered for shore, and the crowds went still, ceasing their marching, lowering their signs, raising their eyes. Battle lines blurred and enemies decamped, standing side by side, for now, in their common wish: that the girl they now knew was flying above them, and her passengers, would find a safe landing.

Now.

"Flory, now."

Nose down, pull back on the throttle. We have to

touch down at the slowest speed possible. That's it. And . . . we're dropping. Keep your eyes on the shoreline, don't watch the water, it'll fool you. Short damn lake, but they said it was long enough, pilots used to land here all the time. With the engine off, of course. Slowest speed possible, right? All right, and lower. That's it. Keep into the wind, it'll slow you down even more. There's the water, wavelets coming straight for you. Water rudders retracted, maximum landing flap now. Close the throttle *now*. Power off. Silence.

Silence. A bird.

And, nose up for the landing flare, don't want the float tips getting buried in the lake. Or us. We're dropping. Nose steady, eyes on the shoreline . . . there! No . . . was that it? A bounce . . . there. There! We're down. The drag of the water on the floats, better than brakes. Slower, slower. We're drifting now. No control. I'm done. We're done. We're down.

"And one, and two, and three, and four . . ."

She saw the Search and Rescue crew launch from the dock. Could hear the sirens now. Police voices shouting through bullhorns. And the cheering. And the applause. Both sides united, for now, by the drama still unfolding before them. And then the rescue crew was there, opening the cockpit door, taking over from Amy, taking the controls, taxiing the plane to the dock. "Nice landing, Miss. You three, that's Jerry, go see him, get yourselves checked over. Your pilot's alive—good job. Can't tell for how long, though. We'll stabilize him, transfer him to an ambulance, get him to hospital. Go, go. It's okay. We got him."

Jane, Amy, and Flory climbed out onto the dock, blinking in the glare of the midday sun and the media cameras. "Enough. Back off, please," said the paramedic named Jerry. "Medical personnel. Clear the way."

Evie came running down the path and out onto the dock. "Are you crazy?" She caught Jane up in a hug and wouldn't let her go. "Are you okay?"

Jane nodded as the paramedics hurried by carrying Ralph on a stretcher. "I am, Evie, and the vaccine is safe, but you'd better call Shelley and tell her to get down here right away." She pointed to the ambulance as it sped away, sirens blaring. "That's her fiancé."

As they made their way up the path, a tall form stood out above the crowds, sleek coif and elegant attire entirely out of place, military posture unmistakable. Avis. Jane pushed past a group of camera techs and threw herself at her friend.

After a long moment, and without a word, Avis steered the three of them firmly away from the cameras and toward the parking lot. Jane felt a sob rising and choked it off. Not here. Not yet. "Into the car, all of you," Avis ordered, her ordinarily stern voice wavering with emotion. "I'm taking you home."

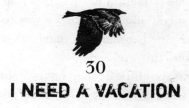

30

I NEED A VACATION

JANE SAT SLOUCHED ON THE LIVING ROOM COUCH, stocking feet up on the coffee table, two furry lumps pinning her midsection to the furniture, staring unseeing at the television screen and listening to the rain. It hammered the roof and ran in mercurial streams down the glass of the big sliding doors that looked out over the lake. It pounded Elfin lake like fists, chopping up the small body of water like the ocean in a storm. It grayed the skies and the air over the lake, and the lake itself, it silvered the windows and colored the room and everything in it, leveling, blanketing, muting. It teemed. And it had not stopped since Jane arrived home.

Another sound had Jane's attention, this one inside the house. It was her mom, moving from room to room, tidying, filing, organizing, puttering. She couldn't remember the last time she'd heard those sounds, the last time she'd been at home with anyone other than Sweet Pea and Minnie for company. It was the holiday Monday of the long weekend, and by some miracle of scheduling, her mom had decided to spend the day away from the restaurant to "get caught up." Jane suspected she might also have found a way to stay home just to make sure her daughter didn't try piloting any more airplanes this weekend.

"How was your little holiday, honey?" she had asked innocently when Avis dropped her at the door.

Jane had exploded then, the fear and strain of the past two and a half days finally catching up with her. Her mom had heard the whole story, at top volume, eyes wide, hands on her heart. Then Jane had rushed past her up the stairs and into the bathroom, slamming the door. She'd stood under a steaming shower, tears mingling with hot water, until some of the tension drained away. Then she'd dressed and slunk to the couch, no idea how to find her way back to "normal."

"Hot cocoa?" Her mom was banging around in the kitchen now, cleaning out cupboards.

Hot cocoa. That sounded normal. "Yeah, um, thanks." Jane leaned back into the pillows and let the sound of the rain wash over her.

Her mom joined her on the couch a few minutes later, setting two steaming mugs and a plate of Cedars leftovers down on the coffee table.

"Nice to have some time together," her mom said through a mouthful of *baklava*. *Don't,* Jane thought to herself. *We can't survive two fights in one day.* But she was exhausted, the terror of the harrowing trip home still holding her neck and shoulders in its grip, and her defenses were down.

"For once," she answered, gulping the hot drink and burning the inside of her mouth.

Slowly, her mom put the rest of her pastry back on the plate. "What's that supposed to mean?"

"It means you're never here," Jane answered, struggling to keep her voice from wobbling and her eyes from tearing up. "Just like always. You're in a different place now, but you're never *here*."

Her mom looked down at her hands, studied her fingernails. "I thought that's what you wanted, Jane," she said quietly. "I thought you wanted me to help dad out with the restaurant. And I *have*. It's going really really well." She paused. "I'm sorry I had no idea what was going on for you this weekend. But Jane, how could I? How could I know something you haven't told me? Is this really all my fault?" She let out a frustrated sigh and buried her face in her hands, clearly exhausted herself. Things *were* going well with Cedars, but it took every ounce of Ellen's and Joe's energies to keep it that way. "What do you want, Jane? A mind-reader for a mother? I have to tell you, I haven't met one yet. More family meetings? A once-a-week mother-daughter night? What would help? For goodness sake, please, tell me. What do you *want*?"

"I want us to be a family again!" Jane wailed, surprising herself with the words. And to her enormous embarrassment, she started to sob like a child. For a moment, all she was aware of was the weight of Sweet Pea and Minnie on her legs and the sound of her own crying. And then her mom's arms encircled her and held her, cats and all. And there it was: all she wanted.

"You know what we Rays need, Janey?" her mom whispered in her ear after a few minutes. She shook her head, and blew her nose loudly into the tissue her mom handed her. *"A real vacation!"*

Jane looked up, hope warring with realism. "Really? But how? You and dad are so busy."

"It wouldn't be for several weeks yet, probably end of August. We'd need to be sure Effie, Elias, and Marcello were ready to handle things on their own," Ellen said pragmatically. "But we could start planning right now! The question is, could *you* get the time off work?"

Jane laughed, having forgotten she was the UWRC's employee as of tomorrow. "I haven't even started yet, and I'll show up on my first day demanding vacation time!" She sniffed and wiped her nose again. "Somehow I think Evie might be okay with that, though."

Her mom smiled. "Next question: where to?"

Jane hesitated for a moment, thinking. Then a memory of jewel colors and raw, magnificent wilderness filled her mind. "I want to go back. Do it right this time. Slow down, see everything."

Her mom nodded, for once hearing everything Jane didn't say. "The Rockies?"

"The Rockies."

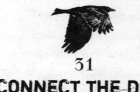

31
CONNECT THE DOTS

L ATE TUESDAY AFTERNOON, when Jane, Amy, and
Flory met at the Shack to compare notes on their
first day of work, they hugged like long-lost relatives.
The previous three days had been so intense that thirty-
six hours apart had felt like forever. Gathering around
the old wooden table and fortifying themselves with
pitchers of lemonade and plates of thick-sliced watermelon, they relived the whole adventure again from
beginning to end. Although they'd been together the
entire time, there were parts each girl had lived through
in her own way, and now was their chance to tell the
others, *This is what it was like for me.* For once, Amy
had no urge whatsoever to exaggerate her version of the
story. It was already so extraordinary that the weight
of further embellishment threatened to render it utterly
unbelievable to anyone she might tell. Truth, this time,
was stranger than fiction.

Ralph Mailer had survived three hours of heart
surgery and was recovering in intensive care. Evie
and Shelley had arranged to trade jobs for a week so

Shelley could be close by, and she'd already stopped at the MacGillivray house to present Amy with a huge bouquet of flowers. She'd been unable to speak, even to say thank you, but Amy hadn't minded a bit.

Buster, too, had lived, turning the corner shortly after Amy had gone to see him at the vet hospital Monday afternoon. He was weak, and would have to stay indoors for several days, but he was home.

Sated at last with the details of their recent exploits, they moved on to trade stories of first-day outfits, bosses and co-workers, and juicy office gossip. Buster lay under the table at their feet throughout, tail whumping companionably on the floor. The rain had stopped but the sun had yet to return, leaving the sky gray, damp, and muggy. Amy had set up an old metal fan in the corner, but it seemed to do little more than push the heat from one end of the room to the other.

"She is *so* totally into him, but I can tell it's not mutual," Amy was saying of two other interns at the lab as she wiped watermelon juice from her chin. She leaned in and lowered her voice to a whisper, although there was no one else around to hear: "In fact, I'm almost positive I caught him checking out my hair."

Jane and Flory burst into laughter. "Amy, *everybody* checks out your hair," Jane teased her. "I see *old ladies* checking out your hair when we go to the park. It's . . . well, it's alarming, is what it is. At times, I mean. No offense." Flory muffled another guffaw. "Ben doesn't have anything to worry about with this guy, does he?"

Amy stuck out her tongue by way of response, then retreated to the computer to answer a ping—"from Benoît, *naturellement!*" Soon she was giggling and typing furiously. Jane and Flory rolled their eyes at one another, grinning, and then settled back in their chairs to wait for the flurry of passion to spend itself.

"You must have had a hero's welcome at the wildlife center this morning, Jane," Flory said as she pulled a stack of shopping magazines from her bag. She'd assembled a very versatile work wardrobe to carry her through the summer, but she was still lacking a few key accessories. "How did the first vaccinations go?"

Amy spun in her chair. "Hey, yeah! Tell all!"

Jane laughed out loud at the contrast between her friends' vision of her first day of work and reality. "Well . . ." she paused dramatically, "first of all, Daniel and Shelley administered the vaccinations. *I,* on the other hand, cleaned poopy cages for the patients in the care room. *Then* I hosed down poopy kennels outside on the wash deck, and then, let me think, oh yeah, then I scrubbed poop off towels and kennel pads and did some laundry, and while the machines were going, I headed outside and scraped poop off the cement floor of the pigeons' aviary. By then it was lunch time—and yes, Amy, I washed my hands first." Amy hooted and applauded. "After lunch," Jane continued, "we scrubbed down all of the outbuildings and painted over the graffiti. This guy who owns a local glass shop came by, said he saw the news last night and wanted to donate all new windows for the Care Center"—Jane paused to clear her throat—"so we took measurements for those. And we all kept our timers with us the whole time, since we still had to feed the babies every fifteen minutes and the fledges every forty-five. Then the evening volunteers arrived at 4:00 p.m., thank goodness, to start the final rounds of cleaning and diets. So yeah, basically a typical day." She slumped in her chair, thinking for the hundredth time how well she'd sleep that night.

"Business as usual, hey, Jane?" Amy said, grinning at her lifelong friend. Only Plain Jane could trade glory for animal droppings and be happy about it.

"Pretty much," Jane nodded thoughtfully. "But you know, that's what was so special about today. It *was* business as usual!" She sat up straight, realization dawning fully for the first time. "No protestors, no signs. Everybody's car in the parking lot when I arrived. No tension, no death threats in the inbox, no worry lines on anybody's face." In fact, the staff had fairly floated around the Care Center, administering meds, supervising admissions, accepting countless donations, and cheerily seeming to disobey the laws of gravity.

"The other thing," she added, her throat tightening a little as she remembered, "was overhearing Anthony admit a crow that had hit this lady's window. He said to her, 'We'll vaccinate it against West Nile Virus and treat it for head trauma, ma'am. This bird will have every chance.'" She looked up into her friends' eyes then, her own eyes brimming with tears. Every chance. No guarantees, not even with the vaccine, but still, every chance. Every animal deserved that.

Jane recalled that the woman had asked anxiously whether West Nile Virus had arrived yet in Cedar's Ridge. "Not as far as we know, ma'am," had been Anthony's answer.

"Hey, Ame," she said nonchalantly, "did you do any actual work at that lab of yours today?"

Amy had turned back to the computer screen and was scanning Ben's latest message. "Hmm?" She giggled and then gasped. "Benoît Tremblay! You're making me blush! What's that, Jane? Ohhh . . . did I get some test results, do you mean?" Amy spun around and reached for something in her satchel. Jane felt her heart start to race. "Nope!" Amy said, disappointingly. "Thursday, I'm hoping. But I did get this today!" She handed Jane an official-looking document on Cedar's Ridge Veterinary Hospital stationery. "Buster's toxicology report. It took Dr. Reid forever to figure out what was wrong with him, poor little buddy. And no wonder!"

Jane reached for the report with one hand and bent over to scratch the soft tuft of sandy hair between Buster's ears with the other. The gentle old retriever closed his eyes and pressed his head into her hand, transported. *Funny how something as small as a pat on*

the head or a hug can make you feel like you're in heaven,
she thought. Of course, they always said a brush with
death does wonders for your appreciation for life.

Clinical Records and Toxicology Report for Buster MacGillivray

History/Presenting Problem:

One-week history of vomiting, diarrhea,
poor appetite with progressive signs of
lethargy/depression. One-day history of
muscle tremors, also progressive. Bloodwork
and radiographs performed by Dr. Reid
revealed no diagnostic abnormalities.

Physical Exam Findings:

Thin body condition, lethargy, slow heart
rate, poor muscular coordination, mental
activity normal but subdued, generalized
muscle tremors present during examination,
increased respiratory effort. Temp = 103.46

Assessment:

Concerned regarding possible toxicity
(strychnine, metaldehyde, organophosphate
(OP), chocolate, other) vs other metabolic/
organic disease.

Treatment:

Repeat bloodwork, place on IV fluids,
induce general anesthesia, evacuate stomach
contents via large-bore gastric tube

(collect contents and send for toxicology screen), administer activated charcoal to bind toxin and prevent further absorption. Once awake, consider atropine/valium as needed to control clinical signs.

Toxicology:

Multiple fur samples and 70ml of gastric contents analyzed. Organophosphate (OP) compounds consistent with agricultural pesticide isolated from both.

Home Care Instructions:

Buster's clinical signs, response to therapy, and toxicology findings are consistent with OP toxicity due to both oral and dermal exposure. He has responded well. Provided there is no further exposure, his prognosis is good.

Jane was staring at the toxicology report but seeing the giant billboard just outside of Hope, the one where half the slats had turned, presenting a picture of the waterslide park, and the other half were stuck, still advertising designer men's underwear. She could practically hear the gears grinding. Poison. Charcoal. She'd spent half her time at the UWRC these past two months helping Daniel try to save poisoned birds. This report was ringing bells. Was there a connection?

"Jane, what is it?" Flory was eyeing her closely. "Is

there something suspicious in the report?"

At that, Amy turned around again, Ben abandoned for the moment. Jane handed the report to Flory without a reply and then said, "Amy, where do you walk Buster?"

"Huh?"

"Humor me."

"Oh. Well, usually the trails around Elfin, that's our regular route, although at least once a week we hike to the top of the hill and walk the length of the ridge. There's a nice, big pond up there for you to swim in, isn't there, boy?" Buster padded over at the sound of Amy's voice and flopped down on her feet. "On our ambitious days, we circle the whole top of the ridge, past your condos, Flory, the golf course, around the park and the elementary school, and all the way back down."

Jane nodded as Amy talked, trying to visualize the route in her mind's eye. "If only I had a city map . . ."

Flory pulled a black file folder out of her bag and withdrew a slim document folded many times over. "This was part of our welcome package today," she said, opening it out and laying it on the table. It was a map of Cedar's Ridge, four feet by six, created from an aerial photograph. Jane could even see her own house.

"Flory, have you ever considered a second career as a genie?" Amy asked appreciatively.

"Oh, wow, Flor," Jane said, itching to get her hands on the map. "Is it okay if I . . . I mean, what I have in mind is going to kind of . . . wreck it."

Flory held her hands out as if to say, it's all yours.

Jane leapt to her feet, sweeping the map off the table and grabbing a box of push-pins from the computer desk. Stepping behind Amy's lab table, she pinned the map to the wall. "Amy, do you think you could trace out the route you just described?" she asked.

"Yeah, no problem," Amy replied, grabbing a blue marker from the desk and stepping up to the map. "But do you mind telling me why?"

"I . . . actually, I don't know yet," Jane answered, frustrated. She could only see half the picture, couldn't yet imagine the missing bits. Maybe when she was through, she'd have an image of something as innocuous as waterslides or men's underwear. But maybe . . .

Amy marked the route she and Buster followed on their "ambitious days," outlining a shape on the map that resembled an overweight alligator. "Excellent!" Jane exclaimed. "Now, may I make a phone call?"

Amy widened her eyes, looking over at Flory and then back at Jane. "My friend, I think you need to start wearing a mask when you clean cages at the Center," she said in what she obviously thought was a compassionate tone. "You've been inhaling again."

Jane bit her lip, feeling as crazy as she sounded, and glanced over at Flory for reassurance. The small girl quickly scanned Buster's toxicology report again, looked back at the shape on the map, then turned to face Jane. "You call the Center," Flory said, "I'll call the vet." Jane grinned her thanks and pulled the red phone to the table in front of her. Flory punched the number on the report into her cell phone.

"What am I missing?" Amy cried in despair. "Other than the gene for insanity?"

Jane glanced at her watch: already after 5:00 p.m. Would Anthony still be there? Yes! "Anthony, hi, it's Jane. Could you spare me about ten minutes? Ame, red pen." For the next ten minutes, Amy made red dots on the map according to the instructions Jane called out as she talked to Anthony. When Flory flipped her phone closed, she listed five locations, which Amy then marked on the map in green.

"Thanks, Anthony," Jane was saying. "If I come up with anything, you guys'll be the first to know. See you tomorrow."

She cradled the receiver and looked up to find the blue alligator encircled by dozens of red dots and five green ones. There was also a small clump of red dots below and to the left of the alligator—below the ridge and to the east of Elfin Lake—and a few more scattered randomly throughout the ridge.

"*What*," Amy said slowly through clenched teeth, "*in the name of all things holy are we looking at?* My dog almost dies, you two want to play connect the dots, you'd better start EXPLAINING!"

"Poison." Jane went to Amy and took her hand. "Each of those red dots represents an animal that was brought to the wildlife center in the past two months that had to be treated for poison. Or StickiStep," she added. "I asked Anthony for both. See, we always ask people who bring animals to the Center where they found them, so that we can try to release them as close as possible to their home or social group. The information was all there. Just, nobody'd put it together before."

Flory was nodding. "The green ones are domestic animals—four dogs and one cat—that were treated for the same poison as Buster in the past two months. And just think—that's only one vet hospital! There may have been more cases as well, at other clinics!"

Amy stared at the map, disbelieving. "Somebody deliberately poisoned my dog?" she whispered.

Jane shook her head. "Not sure about that yet. Buster's report says 'agricultural pesticide.' It could be some overly ambitious gardener trying to keep his lawns green, or maybe . . ."

"Where does Jake Harbinsale live?" Flory's voice came out sounding thin and strangled. Jane's heart stopped. At first she thought Flory was asking if she knew where Jake was. She'd kept that secret since the night she'd seen him at Cultus Lake, not telling even her best friends. But as she started to breathe again, she realized Flory just wanted to know where the Harbinsale house was located on the map. She took a step closer, finding her own home again and then tracing the lake-shore until she reached . . . the small clump of red dots.

"Here," she said, her own voice catching, her finger on the red circle. "Right here."

Flory raised her hands to her mouth, her face gone completely white. "No," she whispered. "Oh, no. It's the pest-free city."

By the time Flory had finished explaining the situation at City Hall to Amy and Jane, her friends were speechless. "The proposal was defeated five to four at the last vote, but it comes up before Council again at next week's meeting. Rand Harbinsale will probably be spending this Thursday night's meeting trying to sway at least one more council member to vote his way. And if he does . . ." she paused, and looked to the dots on the map, "before summer's through, the whole city will look like that."

Jane broke in: "Flor, did you say the pest-free city thing lost five to four?"

Flory nodded, "That's right . . . Ohhhh!"

"Uncle!" Amy called, raising her hand.

Jane squinted at her legal-minded friend. "Do you think it's just a coincidence?"

"I couldn't say," Flory conceded. "And no way to find out. The votes are secret, of course."

"UNCLE!" Amy shouted. Buster let out a startled "woof."

"Sorry, Ame, Rand Harbinsale's investment club,"

Jane said, realizing belatedly that Amy was keeping up with her leaps of logic about as well as Buster was. "Four city councilors: Rand, Madge Moody, Rishi Parmar, and Buzz Gunnarson. Four councilors vote for the pest-free city. Coincidence?"

"I think not!" Amy exclaimed, catching on.

"Too soon to say," Flory corrected. "We don't have enough information."

"Can we get it?" Jane leaned forward.

Flory nodded. "City Hall has copies of business registrations and officers on file, all public domain. You could get it, too. Anybody could. If their database is in good shape, I should be able to complete a search for those four names. Whatever they're involved in, I'll know by the end of my lunch hour."

Jane nodded. "Whatever you find, can you bring me four copies? No, wait . . . make it five. And Ame? Five copies of Buster's toxicology report, with all your personal info blotted out. Did you take any pictures of him while he was sick?" Amy nodded slightly, recalling her frenzy to capture every last detail and expression of her beloved dog on camera in case he didn't make it. "If you'd feel okay about me using one . . . No? Never mind. Sorry. I shouldn't have asked. So, I'm going to get the examination and treatment records for every single one of those red dots, and photos of the animals, too, if Daniel can make me copies. If this is . . . Flory . . . where did you get those?"

Flory was in the midst of jotting reminder notes to herself on a couple of manila card tags. She looked up sharply, hearing the urgent note in Jane's voice. "These tags, you mean?" She blushed then. "Oh, I'm so ashamed, Jane . . . I stole them from work! It's just that Supplies over-ordered them, so we've all got stacks in our desk drawers to use as scrap, and I thought . . ." She groaned. "See? I *knew* I'd get caught!" She shoved the scribbled notes into the pocket of her bag.

Jane shook her head, perplexed. She hadn't meant to rat Flory out for stealing. It was just that she was sure she'd seen those tags somewhere before. *Yeah, and on the grand scale of importance, that's right up there with remembering to trim Minnie's claws some time this month,* she thought to herself. "Okay, so we're clear? We'll meet back here same time tomorrow and see what we've got." She drained the last of her lemonade. "I'm going for a run. Anybody game?"

"I'll do anything, as long as I can stop thinking now," Amy said drily. Jane grinned and pulled her to her feet.

"I'll pass," Flory said, hastily shoving manila tags into her bag. "I think I had better go to Confession."

32
DINNER DATE

Wednesday after school, Amy laid five copies of Buster's toxicology report on the old wooden table, MacGillivray name and contact information blanked out. Then she placed five copies of a photograph on top of the pile—a tired and emaciated Buster gazing up at the camera from the hearth in the big house, his eyes clouded by pain and medication.

Jane looked up quickly at her friend, her own eyes momentarily clouded by tears. "Ame, are you sure?"

"I don't know what you have in mind, Jane Ray," Amy answered, "but if this picture can help save other animals from going through what Buster did, then use it."

"Thanks," Jane said softly. In turn, she laid out the UWRC case sheets for the wild animals affected by poison and StickiStep between early May and early July—seventy-three animals in all. Daniel kept photo records of all their patients, and had said he could have duplicates of these ones for her by Thursday afternoon.

Flory had been sitting quietly at the table, her bag in her lap, paying close attention to the documents the other girls set out. Now, as they sat down and looked over expectantly at her, she pulled out a thin sheaf of papers and spread them across the table: Exhibits A through Z, ladies and gentlemen of the jury.

"Councilors Rand Harbinsale, Margaret Moody, Rishi Parmar, and Gordon Gunnarson are all significant shareholders in GreenGrow Enterprises Inc.," Flory stated matter-of-factly. "Jane's 'coincidence' of yesterday is coincidence no more. These four are our pest-free city proponents, I am sure."

"GreenGrow?" Jane said slowly. "That doesn't ring any bells, Flor."

"The name of the parent company may not sound familiar," Flory conceded, "but one of its products will. GreenGrow makes StickiStep Pest Repellent."

Jane shook her head in wonder. Although the news was not entirely a surprise—she'd trusted her hunch of yesterday—the thought that all those polluted animals, all those oil-baths, all the costs for their care were the result of this "dream team's" vision for a more livable Cedar's Ridge was almost more than she could believe.

"There's more," Flory interrupted her thoughts. "GreenGrow also manufactures Bug-Off for Lawns and Greens."

A light came on in Amy's eyes. "Bug-Off—that was the chemical analysis City Hall wanted from us in such a big rush today. I worked on that!"

Flory blushed. "I might as well move into the church,

I go to Confession so much these days." She sighed. "It was me who ordered that report—right after I added a few years to my seniority level on the requisition form."

"*And?*" Jane asked, looking back and forth between Amy and Flory.

"Organophosphate-based agricultural pesticide," the two of them said in unison.

"Buster's poison," Jane breathed.

"They tried to kill my dog!" Amy sat back in shock. "They tried to kill my dog!"

Flory shook her head. "No. What happened to Buster, and the other dogs and cat, was an unfortunate—though potentially lethal—by-product of their efforts. Ironically enough, they were trying to kill mosquitoes."

"Have they not heard of a fly swatter?" Amy wailed.

"Not one big enough to keep West Nile Virus out of Cedar's Ridge," Flory replied, utterly serious. "And that was their plan. Look at our map. That pattern touches all the big and little waterways on the ridge—the river, the lake, the tributaries and creeks and ponds, all potential breeding grounds for mosquitoes. They dumped enough Bug-Off in the water to kill every larva for the next hundred years, I'd guess. Not to mention anything that happened to land within a few feet of shore. And if a few crows and pigeons happened to ingest it, well, so much the better. It probably never occurred to them other animals might drink from those waterways, or swim in them." She shuddered suddenly. "Or maybe it did."

"So let me get this straight," Amy held up her hands. "These people are shareholders in this company, which means they make money when that stuff sells, right?"

"Partly," Flory said.

Jane gasped. "Madge Moody owns Cedar's Ridge EarthWorks! She could sell those products in her store, and make money twice!"

"I placed a quick phone call to EarthWorks just this afternoon," Flory said, a small smile of pride on her face. "And guess what their two top sellers are right now?"

"*Already?*" Amy looked confused. "But I thought the pest-free city hadn't come into effect yet."

"It has for Rand Harbinsale," Flory responded grimly, remembering her meeting with him in the office corridor at City Hall. *The Country Club I manage is already a pest-free zone, as is my own home estate.*

"Just how much of these products can one person buy, Flory?" Amy looked disbelieving.

"It all depends on who that person is buying *for*," Flory said shrewdly.

"Cedar's Ridge Golf & Country Club!" Jane fairly shouted.

"*And* City Parks," Flory finished, stunning them both. "He's been requisitioning the stuff in anticipation of winning the vote."

"So let me get this straight," Amy said for the second

time, as overwhelmed as Jane was by the picture Flory was painting for them. "Rand Harbinsale is using other people's money to buy this stuff—and in the case of City Hall, before he even has approval—and he and his cronies make money every time he does it. Have I got that right?"

"Essentially," Flory nodded. "He's using Club and taxpayers' money to fund his pest-free city scheme, put money in his friends' pockets, and make himself rich as a shareholder! Yep, you've got it right."

Amy whistled. "Nice!"

"Amy!" Flory tsked disapprovingly.

"What?" the mischievous redhead winked at Jane. "You have to admit, the scheme has its merits."

"Well, I guess so, if you're a sociopath," Flory sniffed, clearly spotting a second candidate for Confession.

"Now, Jane," she continued. The others stared at her. Surely there couldn't be more. "Are you sitting down?"

Jane looked back at her friend, one eyebrow raised, certain melodrama had finally gotten the best of her. The three of them had been sitting together at the table for the past half hour. Flory grinned sheepishly and pressed on.

"I found one more business association for Rand Harbinsale, something that I think will come as a bit of a shock . . ."

"SeaKing."

It was Flory who looked shocked. "How did you

know?" She glanced over at Amy, who simply shrugged, completely surprised as well. "Yes! He was the majority shareholder in SeaKing Shipping Pacific. He lost a huge amount of money when the company folded, which probably explains why he's 'working' so hard to make it back now. Jane, how did you know?"

"I just guessed," Jane explained lamely, thinking of her promise to Jake.

"Soooo . . ." Amy interjected, sensing her friend didn't want to be pressed, "what exactly do we do with all this damning evidence, Your Honor?" She looked quizzically at Flory, and then flattened a hand on top of Buster's photos. "And what's all this stuff got to do with it?"

"Well, ladies," Jane responded, a playful note in her voice, "I was hoping you might be free for dinner tomorrow night. My treat. I was thinking maybe Cedars? Around nine-ish? You know, just after the Council Meeting lets out."

Amy and Flory stared at each other, eyes wide, and then turned to stare at Jane. "Ambush?" Flory whispered, a hand over her mouth. Jane nodded. "Time to give the foursome a taste of their own medicine."

"Sneaky, underhanded, dirty fighting," Amy said thoughtfully. "I like it!"

Jane grinned at her two best friends. "See you here, same time tomorrow."

33
NEW MENUS FOR CEDARS

J ANE WAS LATE. "Sorry, guys," she said breathlessly, dropping five Cedars menus onto the wooden table. It was almost six o'clock now, she'd finished work at 4:00, and in between she'd been to five other places all over the city: Cedars to clear her plan with her mom and dad and pick up her parents' car; the Harbinsale home to deliver Jake's message to his mom when she knew for sure Rand would be at City Hall; her doctor for a follow-up checkup; EarthWorks; and downtown to Stanley Park to take one last photo for tonight.

She and her mom and dad had huddled together in the kitchen at Cedars as she tried to explain her plan and convince them that cornering four prominent members of City Council in their restaurant was a perfectly reasonable idea. Her parents had been hell-raisers in their day, and she'd been sure they'd welcome another chance to shake up the establishment. Instead, her dad's face creased with concern, and her mom shook her head. "This could ruin us, Jane," she said frankly. "I'm sorry. I can see you feel strongly about this, but we can't afford to take the chance, not after all we've been through to get the business off the ground. If you're wrong, it would most certainly put us under. But it wouldn't stop there. We could be sued. Blacklisted. We'd never be able to open another restaurant, or any other business, for that matter." She shook her head again. "It's too big a risk." Her dad's silence had served only to strengthen her mom's position.

Jane had pulled a folder from her knapsack then, and handed it to them: copies of every statistic and report and photograph she and Amy and Flory had looked at over the past two days, even the map. Together, her parents had turned the pages, slowly at first, then faster as the import of what they were seeing sank in. Finally, her dad looked up, disbelief mingled with disgust. "Is this all for real?"

"Joe . . ." her mom laid a hand on his arm.

Jane nodded.

"Ellen, I can't stomach this, and I'd be surprised to think you could, either!"

"I can't, Joe, but that's got nothing to do with the restaurant, with our family's livelihood . . ."

"I know you're trying to protect us, Ellen, but there comes a time . . . For heaven's sake, if we let those people eat here after tonight, we're saying this is okay!" He brandished the folder in the air like a flag. "So this plan of Jane's causes the four of them to lose their appetites, so be it. If the restaurant's doing as well as I think it is, we don't need crooks for patrons!" Finished, he slammed the folder down on the chopping block and crossed his arms, staring defiantly at his wife.

To Jane's utter surprise and mortification, her mother grabbed her father by the shoulders and kissed him passionately. "Oh, for . . ." she muttered as the seconds ticked by. "So . . . um . . . hello? Right, so is that a yes?"

Ellen and Joe burst out laughing then, and leaned forward to draw her into their embrace. "It's a good thing," Ellen said, brushing Jane's hair from her face, "that we're all equally crazy. Because tonight could go very very badly. And if it does, we will *all* have to live with the consequences."

Joe grabbed a cleaver and a sharpener from the knife block and grinned like a cartoon villain as steel blade rang against rough metal. "Bring it on!"

"Some date you are, Jane Ray," Amy said, lifting a menu from the table now, the little silver trees of the Cedars logo glinting against the black background. "I thought you were taking us for dinner. What're we doing now, ordering in? Heyyyy . . . does that dreamy Marcello do the deliveries?" She flipped open the menu to make her selection, and started when she discovered that all the plastic page protectors inside had been emptied of their usual fare of appetizers, mains, and desserts.

"N'uh-uh," Jane replied, laying out stacks of case sheets, reports, and photographs in a particular order on the table. "We're inserting today's 'fresh sheet!'"

"Assembly line?" Flory queried, picking up on what Jane had in mind.

Jane nodded. "How about you sort, Amy and I'll stuff."

"How about Flory sorts, *you* stuff, and Amy steals fresh-baked brownies from Mama MacGillivray's kitchen?" Amy asked, already lifting the trap door.

"Mmm," Jane replied. "Excellent idea. Dinner could be . . . late tonight."

Amy descended the stairs into the underground tunnel, and Jane followed behind her, offering to help carry things back from the house. When the trap door closed above her and the tunnel went black, she whispered tentatively into the murk, "Ame?"

"Yeah?" came the reply from a short distance up the tunnel.

"Did you get those test results?" There was a long pause. "Whether you're nodding or shaking your head, Ame, you need to know that I can't see you."

"Oh, right. Yes. Yes we did. You were right, Jane. It'll be in Saturday's news."

Jane stood on the bottom stair and listened to her friend's footsteps fade away in the darkness.

34

A TASTE OF THEIR OWN MEDICINE

JANE, AMY, AND FLORY WATCHED NERVOUSLY from the back hallway as Effie greeted the four City Councilors at the door and showed them to their regular booth at the back of the restaurant. "I'm certain we sold Oberlin on it, aren't you?" Rand Harbinsale was shouting heartily and slapping Rishi Parmar and Buzz Gunnarson on the back. "Next week's a shoe-in!" The girls looked at each other, eyebrows raised. The Councilors were convinced they'd be voting in a pest-free Cedar's Ridge at the next City Council meeting.

Jane noticed they all sat in the same positions at the table as they had last time she was here. She watched closely as Effie handed them their menus—the one on top to Rand Harbinsale, as her dad had instructed—and Elias brought them their usual drinks. Unless she was mistaken, Madge Moody was drinking a Shirley Temple. The four chatted a while longer, clearly heady with anticipated victory. And then . . .

Moody was first to open her menu. She made a sound like a small owl, a tiny hoot that sent the three girls into paroxysms of stifled laughter and caused her companions to reach for their own menus. "Something good in the specials list tonight, Madge?" Harbinsale inquired jovially. "I could really go for a-ag-agghhh!"

"What was that, Rand?" Buzz inquired obsequiously. "I didn't quite catch that. I'll split an appie with you if you don't think you can finish oh my heavens to Betsy I think my vertigo is acting up has anyone got a valium?"

"What are you all to be getting so excited about?" Parmar asked with a chuckle. "I always order my same exact thing but I can't help myself looking every time at all the almighty gods and goddesses I knew we should have gone to the curry place tonight!"

The girls were choking on laughter, shaking as they tried to keep quiet enough to stay close to the action without being overheard. The councilors' table had gone silent, four faces turned a mottled gray, as each of them started at the first page and worked their way from the front of the menus all the way to the very back.

The formal proposal originally tabled with Cedar's Ridge City Council, calling for a pest-free city.

The business registration documents for GreenGrow Enterprises Inc., specifying StickiStep and Bug-Off as subsidiary products and listing major shareholders in the company. The names Gordon Gunnarson, Randall Harbinsale, Margaret Moody, and Rishi Parmar were highlighted in yellow.

A list of every animal brought to the Urban Wildlife Rescue Center to be treated for StickiStep or for poisoning since May, along with a tally of the costs for their care, and the numbers that had not survived.

Photos of the worst cases—birds with their wing feathers matted and torn, toes cemented together, beaks glued shut from trying to free themselves from the deadly trap.

The map, showing the location where each polluted and poisoned animal had been found, their numbers concentrated around the Cedar's Ridge Golf & Country Club and Rand Harbinsale's home.

Buster's photo, and his toxicology report, naming the poison that almost killed him.

The provincial lab's workup on Bug-Off, matching the poisonous compound in the pesticide to the one named in Buster's report.

Five murdered crows laid side by side on the UWRC's examination table, manila tags tied to their legs, scrawled threats easily readable in the photograph.

And in Rand Harbinsale's menu only, a list of the SeaKing Shipping Pacific shareholders, Rand's name at the top, and a photograph of Vancouver's mermaid, the site of the now-defunct SeaKing visible in the background, on the far side of the Inlet. The mermaid had "witnessed" an attack on Jane that almost cost her her life. Perpetrated by SeaKing's Belinda Lee, she was sure. Initiated by Rand Harbinsale? She would never have proof. There was only the silent statue.

The four councilors reached the end of their menus, and still they sat, unmoving, staring at the pages, speechless.

"Why don't they say something?" Flory whispered.

"Like what," Amy hissed back, "four Hail Marys and a Glory Be?"

"Maybe they need time to let it all, uh, soak in," Jane suggested.

"Maybe they're trying to figure out how to make themselves invisible so they can get out of here!" Amy spluttered.

"Actually," Flory broke in, "I don't understand why they haven't already left!"

"I don't think they can," Jane answered.

"Paralyzed with guilt?" Amy scoffed in a stage whisper. "Not likely. Not those four. They don't have one complete conscience between them. Yeah, I don't get it either. If I was caught red-handed like that in a public place, I'd be outta here fast enough to break down your dad's front door."

Jane looked up then at her two best friends. "I wanted to make sure they stuck around long enough to appreciate all our hard work." A wicked sparkle lit her eyes. "I think they might be here a while yet—I sprayed StickiStep on their seats!"

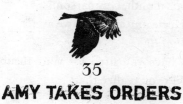

35
AMY TAKES ORDERS

"H I THERE! My name's Amy and I'll be your server tonight! May I take your order?" Amy stood by the Councilors' table, pad and pen poised in her hands, a wad of gum in her mouth, an all-too-genuine grin splitting her face. Jane and Flory muffled squeals in the back hallway. Amy had grabbed an apron from the hook, tied it around her waist, and barged into the restaurant before they could stop her. "Will the Councilors be eating crow tonight?"

"Is this some kind of a sick joke?" It was Rand Harbinsale who spoke, his voice low and menacing, his eyes boring into Amy's. "Where in hell is Effie?"

Amy's grin never wavered. "I'm new! This is my section now." She chewed hard on her gum and returned his murderous gaze. "And Effie's not in hell, mister. But then, I guess you of all people would know that, wouldn't you?" She glanced pointedly at the menu in his hand, and then met his eyes again, daring him to protest any further.

"This is an outrage, you little . . ."

"Shut your mouth, Gunnarson."

"Do you have *any* idea who we are?"

"I said, *shut it!*"

"I could have you fired for your insubordination, young lady, do you realize that?"

"SHUT . . . UP!"

"Randall, calm down," Madge Moody simpered, baring her tiny teeth in a sort of smile. "This is just some juvenile prank. We all need to calm down. We need to think. And perhaps we're not in the mood for Mediterranean food tonight after all." She waggled her sausage curls urgently toward the front door.

"Subtle, Moody," Rand spat back. "You want to leave, leave. You want to stay, you can shut up, too."

"You are not to be telling her to be shutting up!" Rishi Gill brandished his menu menacingly in Rand's face.

"Easy, darling, er, Mr. Parmar. Ahem!" Madge blushed from her neck to the roots of her sausages. "I know when I've overstayed my welcome." Her honeyed voice turned harsh. "You would all be wise to follow me out that door this instant."

She made to rise and, ever the gentlemen, Rishi and Buzz rose first to acknowledge her departure. There was a frightful tearing sound as they left the seats of their pants in the booth. Gunnarson, it seemed, was a boxers man. Parmar preferred briefs.

Madge Moody, already on her way up, failed to halt

her trajectory in time and lost her elastic-waist flowered skirt to the booth. Whereas the men had the dignity of their pant fronts, Madge's scarlet panties, garter belt and black lace hose were now on full display to every patron in Cedars Mediterranean Café.

Amy uttered a low whistle. "It's always the quiet ones."

Rand Harbinsale stared in astonishment at his fellow councilors, then threw back his head and laughed. And laughed and laughed. Amy wondered if he would ever stop. When he finally did, she wondered whether he'd ever bring his head back to vertical again. Apparently, Jane had really spread that StickiStep stuff around. Rand's hair was glued to the top of the booth, forcing his gaze to the ceiling. His notorious temper soon followed it through the roof.

"Get . . . me . . . the hell . . . OUT OF HERE!" he roared. Flailing his arms, he accidentally brushed one of Buzz Gunnarson's naked thighs and screamed as though he'd been burned.

"What in heaven's name is going . . ." Joe Ray stopped short, not at all sure where to look, and momentarily stunned by the all too apparent success of the girls' plan. "Councilors!" he cried, as though he'd been waiting for his cue all along. "In a public place! In *my* restaurant!" Joe clenched his fists as mirth threatened to bubble up through the mock outrage. "What you people do in private is your business, goodness knows, but take it out of here! Now!" He reached into his apron pocket, pulled out an old Polaroid camera, and snapped a photo for good measure.

"Now!" Amy squealed, grinning and chomping on her gum. "And take that filthy slipcover with you!"

"We . . . we were just leaving," Madge Moody murmured as she slithered down the booth and back into her skirt. She reached up with both hands as if to pull Rishi and Buzz back into their seats, then thought better of it, and barked, "Sit!" They sat. Examining the fabric they were stuck to, she realized for the first time theirs was the only booth in the restaurant with a removable slipcover. She glared up at Amy, who popped a bubble and smiled.

"Will that be take-out, Councilor?" she winked.

"Left," Madge hissed. "On three. One, two . . ."

It's like a centipede, Amy thought, head tilting as she watched the eight-legged creature launch into a tap dance routine beneath the table. *A centipede with four heads, both types of gonads, and no brain.* She snorted, almost swallowing her gum.

At last, the four councilors extracted themselves from behind the booth and stood uncertainly in the middle of the restaurant, bent at the knees and again at the hips where StickiStep held them to the stiff fabric. Rand had an extra bend at the neck that left him unable to see where he was going, and so was forced to hold Buzz's hand as they shuffled toward the front door. The laughter of the other patrons had long ago drowned out the music, and Elias could barely keep up with the drink orders. No one had seen a show this good in years.

"I had no idea Cedars did dinner theatre!" one woman shouted to her husband over the noise.

"I had no idea our City Councilors had thespian tendencies!" he replied, clinking her glass with his own.

From her vantage point in the hallway, leaning against Flory as they collapsed in fresh gales of laughter, Jane decided that the bent foursome and their port-a-booth looked like part of a midway ride that had been flung loose mid go-around. As they spun this way and that, seeking the door and finally squeezing themselves out into the night, she thought, *The Tilt-A-Whirl. Or maybe the Hellevator. Or no, maybe my favorite—the Mad Mouse.*

36
TAKE-OUT AND DELIVERY

AMY AND FLORY MUNCHED GREEDILY on stuffed grape leaves and eggplant casserole, hand-feeding Jane from their containers as she drove. "Mmm . . . thanks! Hey, do you ever think to yourself, that was the funniest thing that'll ever happen in my life and nothing can top it?"

"No," Amy said through a mouthful of food as she grooved to the radio. "You ain't seen nothin', girly-girl! I'm jus' gettin' started! Yeah, *watch out!*"

"You scare me, Amy," Jane said, straighfaced.

"'S why you love me, baby!" Amy crowed.

Flory started to giggle and threw herself against the back seat, arms wide. "Just think . . . we still have the whole summer ahead of us!"

"Yeah, Jane," Amy chimed in again. "Still time to find a boyfriend!"

"Oh, for . . . Flory, please tell me you've got that fifth menu back there?" Jane glanced in the rear-view mirror.

"Mmpf!" Flory responded from the back seat, eating again.

"Sheesh!" Amy said disgustedly, popping a grape leaf into her own mouth when Jane didn't take it right away. "All work, no play. You know what they say, keener!"

"We're not finished the mission!" Flory chastised her, wiping her mouth neatly with a paper napkin. "Work first, play later. So Jane, the menu goes in the envelope," she said, licking the gummed flap and sealing the package. Then she pulled a marker from her bag and held it poised over the envelope: "And who is the lucky recipient?"

Jane turned right into the parking lot of the *Cedar's Ridge City Herald* and pulled up to the front entrance. "'City Hall reporter' should do it," she said. "There's the night drop box by the far door, Flory. Do it quick, and then let's get out of here before anybody sees us. I've had enough notoriety for one summer."

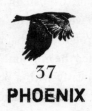

37
PHOENIX

CEDAR'S RIDGE CITY HERALD
West Nile Virus Leaps Rockies, Lands Hard
Saturday, July 8

PROVINCIAL HEALTH ALERT—Health authorities have announced that West Nile Virus has definitively arrived, and warn residents to take all necessary precautions to prevent exposure to the potentially deadly disease. Provincial labs first detected the virus in a corvid captured by the Urban Wildlife Rescue Center in Cedar's Ridge. The crow died in care shortly thereafter. Although it is the only animal in the province so far to test positive, health authorities have also confirmed the first human death by the virus, of one elderly Fraser Valley resident. A second case has been confirmed, in a Cedar's Ridge teen who is believed to have contracted the virus while in the Fraser Valley region. The teen recovered fully and is now immune from the virus for life.

West Nile Virus first arrived in North America in . . .

It was Saturday night at Cultus Lake, the second weekend in July. The cottages were filled with cheery, relaxed holidaygoers, the lake was busy with swimmers, paddle boaters, and windsurfers, and everywhere the smells of woodsmoke and fire-cooked food filled the air. Jane, Amy, and Flory had a small campfire to themselves, well off the path and tucked away in the woods. It was their first moment alone since Thursday evening. Each girl had spent Friday night with her family, and then arrived at Cultus at different times this afternoon. In forty-eight hours, a lot could happen—and usually did.

The resignations of four Cedar's Ridge City Councilors had been eclipsed by the announcement of the arrival of West Nile Virus. Every media outlet in the province had carried the news. "You think that's drama?" Amy bellowed, slathering herself in mosquito repellent til she shone. "I'll give you drama, people. You can keep your double-dealing fraud, your dirty politics, your corporate greed, and your fatal diseases! They are nothing, nothing, you hear me?"—Jane and Flory smiled surreptitiously at one another; there was no chance of *not* hearing the bellowing redhead once she found her soapbox— "*nothing* compared to my *brother* showing up for *dinner* last night with his *girlfriend* to announce to Clan MacGillivray that he will *not* be going to university to study engineering after all"—she paused here to breathe—"but has decided instead to go back to the land, not that he was ever *on* the land, mind you, but *back* to the land to become an *organic farmer*, not for the summer, oh no, but for the *rest* of his lettuce-picking *life!*" Spent, she plopped herself down in a lawn chair and stared at the others.

Flory's hands covered her mouth, and the eyes that peeked over them were wide with amazement. "Mike's quitting school?" she squeaked. "Oh, Amy . . . what did your mom say?"

Amy snorted. "You know her! In the MacGillivray household, school rules. As long as you're going to school, you get free room and board. No school, no gruel. From now on, Mike's on his own. As far as my parents are concerned, he's turned his back on a major scholarship and a chance for a real career. They can't figure out where they went wrong, you know, how they managed to raise such a delinquent. And while they mull that over, they're not actually speaking to him." Amy shook her head. "So now Mike figures if he's gotta pay room and board anyway, he may as well live at the farm where he's going to be studying, which is on some island somewhere off the coast. He'll work this summer at the same farm as last year, here in the Valley, and then in September, he's gone."

"So will he, uh, move in with Katrina for the summer?" Flory asked, with a quick glance at Jane.

Amy bolted out of her chair again. "Oh, noooo! That

was the sucker punch! I honestly think he brought her along for support, figuring she'd tell him his plan was fabulous and tend whatever wounds he might have after battling it out with my parents." She shook her head and cringed. "After the big scene with my parents, the two of them take off to the den. Next thing I know, she's walking out the door, and he's locking himself in his room. I haven't had a chance to really talk to him yet. All I know is, it's over."

Flory moaned sympathetically, her hands over her heart. Suddenly, both she and Amy noticed that Jane had remained strangely still and silent throughout the entire tale. About to sit down again, Amy leapt up once more and shot an accusatory finger into Jane's face: "Aha! I thought so! You *knew!* You knew all about this farmer stuff all along, didn't you? And you never said a *word!*"

Jane gave a slight nod, biting her lip. She'd known about the "farmer stuff," yes, but not what Mike would decide. Not until this moment. And she'd never really believed that his decision would cost him his relationship with Katrina. "I'm sorry, Ame," she said, looking over at her friend. "I really am. I sometimes think . . . I would have preferred not to know anything at all than to wait all this time for him to find the courage to finally say something. It's not some sudden, flighty decision, if that's any consolation. He's been thinking about this since last fall. But it wasn't my secret to tell."

Amy stared at her friend for a long moment, eyes narrowed. Finally, she slouched into her chair and sat, legs splayed, staring at the fire. "Fair enough. Geez. No-good, secret-keeping trustworthy freak of a best friend," she muttered.

Flory giggled at that. "At least we know our secrets are safe with Jane."

"Our lives," Amy said quietly, and for a moment, as the fire crackled cheerily, they all relived that final descent in the floatplane.

"Speaking of secrets," Amy said then, back at full volume, "how about we finally get this underground, unspoken crush you have on my unkempt, unsupported, beet-picking, dirt-poor brother out into the open, hey? Hey, Jane Ray? Think about it. He's fair game now, now that Katrina's out of the picture!" It was Jane's turn to gasp. "Oh, don't be all coy with us. You're *mad* about the boy!"

Jane felt her face flush hot as flames and looked quickly to Flory for support. She found none. "It's true, Jane," Flory chided her softly. "Everyone sees it but you."

Jane fumed. She couldn't believe it. Both her friends had turned on her in an instant. The ambush at Cedars on Thursday was nothing compared to this.

"Every time someone mentions his name," Amy chimed in, "or for that matter any word with the long 'I' sound in it, your pupils dilate and your face flushes, much like now . . ."

"And your voice softens and you get this wobbly little smile on your face," Flory added.

"Basically," Amy concluded, "it's disgusting!"

"What is disgusting, *ma petite?*" Ben Tremblay had materialized out of the darkness and placed his hands on Amy's shoulders. Before she had a chance to answer, he bent down and drew her into a long kiss. *If blushing and smiling are disgusting, what is* that? Jane thought, still furious with her friend for making these ridiculous accusations about Mike. The joke was getting old, frankly.

Mark Co wasn't far behind Ben, and he crossed the circle and sat himself at Flory's feet. She beamed, and ran a hand through his hair for a minute, then bent to whisper something in his ear. He nodded, rose to his feet, and lifted Flory to hers. "We have arrived to escort you ladies to the dance," he said, winking and bowing. "Jane, will you join us, please? I happen to know for a fact that there are a number of fair princes at the ball tonight who will be hoping for a dance with a certain Cinderella!"

Jane smiled, struck as always by his thoughtfulness. *Hang onto that one, Flory,* she thought. Out loud, she said, "Thanks, Mark. Go ahead. I'll catch up with you in a few minutes."

As the two couples left the little clearing, Jane could just make out soft strains of music drifting back from the Community Hall. Soon, though, the woods closed around her once more, enveloping her with their own subtle music—the breeze playing over the lake and through the trees, the gentle lap of waves on the lakeshore, the chirrup of crickets, and the crackle of the fire. An owl called from high in a nearby tree, and as if in response a squeaking scurry of bats darted past, making for the safety of a roost on the far side of the wood. She heard the soft warbles and caahs of crows calling to one another as they settled for the night and thought of another crow, and another night.

She'd stopped by the Mountainview Country Club that afternoon. The Crone's trailer had been overtaken by a family with two small children—Audrey's grandchildren, Jane was almost sure. They'd painted the trim a different color, assembled a swing set on the front lawn, gotten rid of the pretty water garden. *Just as well,* she thought as she waved goodbye to the security guard. *Where you look for her you will not find her.*

The Harbinsale cabin was still boarded up and a For Sale sign sprouted crookedly from the overgrown lawn. Rand had clearly lost no time in trying to liquidate his remaining assets. But the rumors of ghosts had lingered even after Jake and Bobby had left. If anything, they'd become more persistent. *Could be a tough sale,* she thought, and wasn't sorry. She remembered her autumn self hoping and planning to spend this summer with Jake Harbinsale. They hadn't even made it to winter.

And summer, it seemed, had had her own ideas.

In utter disregard for dates and astronomical occurrences, summer had begun in her own good time. According to the calendar, she was three weeks overdue, waiting for things to be put in their proper order, put right, before showing her face. And she had arrived today, along with the news of West Nile Virus, on the wings of a bird that had lived its life as a friend and companion to, a scavenger from, human beings since the beginning of time.

Crow had brought a message of danger, to be sure, but not of the doom and death and destruction people had feared. It was their fear that had brought those things, and they had wanted to kill the messenger to quell their fears. Many still would.

All around her now, Jane could hear messengers, each with its own voice, each with its own story, its own medicine. They spoke to her simply because she listened. That's all it took. *How many others listen?* she wondered. *How many others try to understand? Evie, Daniel, Shelley, other rehabilitators, other animal rescuers, scientists, researchers, writers who listen and tell others what they've heard. Are there enough of us? How much time do we have while the small ones still sing, to hear, to learn to interpret, to act—before the messengers themselves disappear?*

Deep in thought, she felt the soft brush of a wing across her shoulders and spun, startled, to find Mike

MacGillivray standing over her, a tentative smile on his face.

"Oh!" she exclaimed softly. "I thought you were a crow!" She blushed then, clenching her fists, vividly remembering the last time she'd compared him to an animal. Looking up at him now, she saw that he'd shed the showy plumage he'd been wearing then and looked himself in an old gray T-shirt and jeans. For the first time, she noticed that the loose, light-brown curls he kept cropped close to his head looped forward in small fringes at his temples, and that his eyes were exactly the same color as the lake after a thunderstorm. *He's beautiful.* The thought shocked her—where had *that* come from? Did this mean Amy and Flory might possibly be *right?*

She was just as shocked to see how terribly sad he looked. His shoulders slumped as though he'd been beaten in a fight and his eyes held none of their usual mischief, even when he laughed, which he did now in response to her crow comment, much to her relief.

"I wish I *was* a crow," he answered, sitting down beside her and speaking to the fire. "I'd fly away from here in an instant, away from the mess I've made. As it is, I'm heading straight back to the city tonight. I only came to . . ." His voice sank to a whisper, and she strained to hear. "How do you do it, Jane?"

Jane bowed her head, thinking of the mess *she'd* made back in the spring and all that had happened as a result. Surely he didn't think she was . . .

"The animal rescues, defying protestors, fighting corrupt politicians, that crazy flight back over the mountains . . ." He tensed suddenly. "Is it worth it?" he asked fiercely. "For all you give up? For all you lose? Wouldn't it be easier just to keep your mouth shut and go along with everything, live the same kind of life everybody else does? Don't you ever just want to stop asking questions? All those inconvenient questions about agribusiness, genetic modification, terminator seeds? Would it *kill* you to just finish school, get a decent job, get married and have kids and move to the suburbs and just enjoy your paycheque?" Jane suppressed a nervous laugh, not sure whether he was talking to her or to himself. His questions sounded like ones his father might have asked him.

"Cash is good, right?" he went on. "And security? The package? I mean, there's no package for wildlife rehabilitators, is there, Jane? No package for organic farmers. There's not even a set path, you know? Do this, turn right there, and bingo, here's your piece of paper, here's your career, here's your gold watch. The whole thing ahead of me is just . . . *dark!*" He reached a hand out in front of him, as if grasping for some imperceptible sign in the night air.

She could feel the weight and warmth of his body near hers, hear his soft, slow breathing, and she knew the exact latitude and longitude of that terrible, lost place. *Crow medicine*. The thought came to her, unbidden, out of the dark. *That's what he's reaching for.* Out loud, she responded, "Dark like a dead end? Or dark like a mystery?"

His breath quickened, and he sat up straighter, considering what she suggested, a possibility that had never occurred to him before. Leaning in so that his shoulder touched hers, he took a slow, deep lungful of air and let it out with a sigh, as though he'd been holding his breath for months.

"You know what?" he asked suddenly, still not looking at her.

"What, Mac?" She waited for it—the unburdening of his struggle with his family, the breakup with Katrina, the decision to disappoint everyone but himself.

He took another deep breath. "You smell like a Jane Ray."

She let out a startled whoop, and then she laughed with him til they were wiping tears from their eyes. He turned then, and gave her a hesitant smile that made her heart leap. Hardly conscious of what she did, she brought her hand to her heart and placed it over that small, sacred space. *Hold on*, she thought. *Hold on.* She rolled her eyes in the dark, feeling like the happiest idiot in the world for discovering she liked Mike MacGillivray the day after his breakup with Katrina and his excommunication from the Clan. *Your timing is impeccable, Ray girl.*

He stood and held out his hand. "Dance?"

For what felt like a very long time, she looked up at him, wanting nothing more at this moment than to feel his arms around her and to have this boy she'd known all her life, her dear friend, solid and warm in her own arms. Then she stood and reached out and took his hand. "Not tonight," she said, wondering if she was quite possibly insane, if she was missing her one chance. *But ask me again,* she thought. *When you've found what you were reaching for.*

The fire was little more than ash, and as they turned to go, a crow made its way across the clearing, hopping through the grass and dirt until it reached the fire pit. Jane would have sworn it was Crow, except that this bird wore no band. Except that Crow was gone. The bird circled the small charred pile cautiously, as though looking for a doorway only it could see. Finding its entrée, it lay itself on the ashes and spread its wings, chortling softly with evident delight. The night had cooled, and the crow was clearly enjoying the intense heat. Whatever feather mites may have been needling it would by now be in search of another home.

Whether it grew uncomfortable, or whether it was simply ready to take flight, the crow suddenly flapped its wings over the ashes causing flames to leap up from dormant coals. The whole clearing glowed orange as flames sent shadows dancing high into the trees, and as Jane and Mike watched, the firebird rose into the air and flew away into darkness.

Jane stared after the vanished phoenix for a long time. Listening. At last she turned to Mike. "Walk me home?" Together, they ambled down the trail toward the cabins, silent, contented with the sounds of dirt and small pebbles crunching beneath their feet, the soft-scented embrace of encircling fir and pine, the grace of distant and familiar stars to light their path.

Flory's Files

For the record, I'd just like to say that I know those two so-called friends of mine roll their eyes every time I open a new file. But let's be honest: what would they do without me? *Or* my files? I'm beginning to think I should have my own series, really.

File #0609001

How to Protect Yourself from West Nile Virus

Minimize contact with mosquitoes! And:

1. Use insect repellents that contain DEET or other approved ingredients.
2. Mosquitoes are most active at dawn and dusk; try staying indoors at these times.
3. Wear protective clothing including long sleeves, pants, and a hat.
4. Install screens on your doors and windows, and check frequently for holes.
5. Mosquitoes lay their eggs in standing water, and it takes only about four days for them to hatch. Even a saucer's worth of water can act as a breeding ground. Empty saucers under flower pots, change water in birdbaths, ponds, and animal bowls often, drain pool covers, and remove debris from your yard that collects water.

Source: The Wildlife Rescue Association of British Columbia website: www.wildliferescue.ca

Crow Facts and Figures

Crows are members of the Corvidae family and are believed to be the most intelligent of all birds. They form tight family units, create and use tools, engage in play, and are reputed to be able to count. The crow has a crackerjack memory: a crow never forgets a food source—or an enemy. The fully grown Northwestern Crow, or *Corvus caurinus*, reaches an average of sixteen inches from the tip of its bill to the tip of its tail, and weighs about 350 grams. Crows in the wild live an average of eight to thirteen years; however, the oldest known wild American Crow was twenty-nine and a half years old!

Crows will eat just about anything and consume eleven ounces of food each day. Although they have a reputation for damaging crops, they often help out farmers by eating harmful insects. Very social animals, crows speak in dialects and depend on interaction with their own kind for their safety and well being. They generally mate for life. Both crow parents take turns sitting on the eggs, and all family members help take care of the young. There are usually four to six eggs in a crow's clutch, and incubation lasts eighteen days. A baby crow is called a simp, and the young fledge at about thirty-five days.

Completely black, crows can easily identify another crow in the distance during the day, and at night, their coloration helps protect them from predators. Confident and aggressive, crows have few enemies. But owls and hawks—and humans who hunt them—are among their most feared predators. Two crows are considered endangered: the Hawaiian crow and the Mariana crow. Quintessential survivors, crows are found everywhere in the world, except for New Zealand, Antarctica, and South America. Perhaps more than any other birds, crows and ravens have been regarded as having deep spiritual significance by cultures around the globe.

What to Do If You Find a Baby Bird

FILE NO.   0609003

Wild bird babies should be with their parents. Animal parents do a much better job of raising their young than humans can. Sometimes, however, a baby has been orphaned, and will need your help.

Nestlings:
- are naked or only partially feathered
- are helpless and unable to stand
- belong in their nest

Okay, so what do I do if I find a nestling?
1. Try to locate the nest, and gently place the bird in it.
2. Watch for the parent. If the parent does not return within two hours, the baby may be orphaned.
3. Call the nearest wildlife rescue center for further instructions.
4. If the nest has been destroyed, you can fashion a makeshift nest. Again, call your wildlife rescue center for help.
5. If you cannot locate the nest, contact your wildlife rescue center and take the baby bird there. The baby cannot survive without a parent and will need the help of a professional rehabilitator.

Fledglings:
- are well feathered and able to stand and hop, but may not be able to fly well
- are out of the nest
- are learning from their parents to fly and find food

I've found a fledgling. Now what?
1. If you see the parent nearby, leave the baby alone.
2. Keep the area safe from cats and other potential predators.
3. If the parent is not nearby, gently place the baby on a low branch and watch from a distance for the parent to return. Again, keep cats away.
4. If the parent does not return within two to three hours, call your wildlife rescue center for advice. The baby may be orphaned and require help.

File #0609004

Crow Expressions

See if you can sprinkle your conversations with these crow-related turns of phrase!

1. The Greeks used to say "Go to the crows!" instead of "Go to Hell!"
2. The Romans might have told you to "pierce a crow's eye" if you were attempting a near-impossible feat.
3. If the Irish said "You'll follow the crows for it," they meant you'd miss something after it was gone.
4. Have you heard the expression, "I have a bone to pick with you"? It used to be, "I have a crow to pick with you!"
5. To find the shortest distance between one place and another, travel "as the crow flies."
6. To "eat crow" is to make up for a mistake in a really unpleasant way.

Check out *Flight or Fight*, the first book in Jane Ray's Wildlife Rescue Series, for more of my files, including:

#0509002—How to Find a Wildlife Rehabilitation Center Near You

#0509004—What to Do If You Find Injured, Orphaned, or Oiled Wildlife

#0509005—How to Make Your Own Animal Rescue Kit

ACKNOWLEDGEMENTS

My humble thanks to the staff and volunteers, and to my Thursday-morning coffee buddies at the Wildlife Rescue Association of BC, for demonstrating crow medicine every day of the year, and to the animals, who call it forth. To Jackie Ward and Liz Thunstrom for reviewing early drafts of the manuscript (during yet another oil spill in Vancouver's Burrard Inlet). Special thanks to Devin Manky and Crystal Simmons for two spectacular covers and the perfect cover girl.

To all of my incredible friends, who support and celebrate me, feed me, nourish me, heal me, and care for me in all ways—I am the richest person I know. Wild congratulations to Kimberley Alcock, who embarks at last on the master's journey; and special thanks to the BC SPCA's Craig Naherniak and Iris Ting for their enthusiastic support of this series; the Baergs in Edmonton, the Da Pontes in Toronto, the Ogilvys in Maple Bay, and the Rays in Victoria for my homes away from home; Janice Beley and Kim Plumley for putting Jane Ray in the media and into schools from coast to coast; Dale at Tyax, Justin Foulkes-Taylor, and Keith Price for the flying lessons; Reid Danielsen, DVM (the *real* hero of the story), for accurately diagnosing and successfully treating Buster MacGillivray; in memory of Tad Dick who always reminded me there was nowhere to go; in memory of Candace Frank, a daughter of the Goddess if there ever was one, who showed me that we are all one; to Mellifluous Hardy for demonstrating yet again what "loyal friend" really means; Nadia Hovan who grabbed the baton and ran, raising hundreds for animals orphaned by Hurricane Katrina; Lisa Jackson who led the way across the invisible border into a Kanata I never knew; Amahra Jaxen for reminding me of what I'm really up to; Henry for the little blue octopus, which I did not use, and for everything else, which I did; Robert Schad and Toronto's EarthRangers for carrying the message to over 50,000 young people every year; Hope Swinimer and Nova Scotia's Hope for Wildlife Society for being the first to give audience to Jane Ray; Naomi Weber, who forgave with such grace, and whose every gift is a treasure; Audrey Bomberry, Brian Maracle, and Bonnie Whitmore, and to the Mi'kmaq of Eskasoni and the Kanyen'keyha of Oshweken for welcoming me as a friend.

Huge thanks to everyone at Whitecap Books, and especially to Rob McCullough for taking the long view; Sonnet Force for her compassionate reading and for making *Crow Medicine* a better book; and Five Seventeen for nailing the cover in one (no fodder for Q&Q this time :). I am grateful to the Canada Council for the Arts for making writing time and single-minded focus possible.

To my family—we chose well—and my Nana, Mary Ogilvy, who had more crow medicine than most, and who tempered it with kindness.

And as always, to all those who protect the small . . .

Thank you.

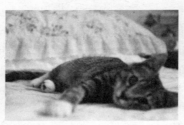

Mouse
(September 15, 1995–August 28, 2006)

A NOTE FROM THE AUTHOR

When I dedicated my first book to Mouse, many of you wanted to know who, exactly, Mouse was. Well, Mouse was my cat. But he was also "the one"—you know, the special someone many of us spend our whole lives waiting for. Mouse was the love of my life.

Mouse was a one-hander when I first met him in October of 1995—a puny grey fur ball who fit in the palm of my hand. He slept between my ear and my shoulder, climbed me like cheap curtains to get to his food before I had a chance to put it on the floor, and fit neatly between an elevator door and the shaft wall with room to turn around and come out again head first. He used up his first life with that trick.

The crack of an egg could bring him from nowhere for a bit of yolk; he reveled in the smells of his garden

from his favorite window ledge; he loved a quiet song sung just for him, to snuggle under the bedcovers and rest his head on the pillow, to ease my workload by stepping into the middle of it and settling in. Christmas was his favorite time of year, with its pine boughs and crackling paper and the whole family together in the house. He was a prodigious hunter in his heyday, and it was with the rare quarry he spared that I made my first trips to the wildlife rescue center where I now volunteer.

You may have noticed that when you learn a new word, suddenly you hear it everywhere, as though your ears have been opened a little bit wider. Loving Mouse opened my eyes to all animals—to the fact that they have needs and wants and feelings like we do, and to the suffering they endure through inadequate legal protection, factory farming, and needless experimentation. Mouse became the reason for my writing, and my inspiration to make our world a better place for animals.

At age five, Mouse was diagnosed with a serious heart condition that meant daily medications and frequent trips to clinics for the rest of his life. At the time, his vet guessed he had about a year to live. Luckily she didn't tell *him* that, or us. He lived another six years, and blessed us every day. I promised him before he died that I would do everything I could to make sure the gifts he gave me and the things he taught me would live beyond us both.